SELF HEALTH GUT GUIDE
DISCOVER THE GUT-BODY CONNECTION TO IMPROVE DIGESTION, SHARPEN YOUR MIND, CREATE LASTING HEALTH, AND FEEL INCREDIBLE EVERY DAY

ELLODY KAMP

© **Copyright 2025 - All rights reserved.**

The content within this book may not be reproduced, duplicated or transmitted without direct written permission from the author or the publisher.

Under no circumstances will any blame or legal responsibility be held against the publisher, or author, for any damages, reparation, or monetary loss due to the information contained within this book. Either directly or indirectly. You are responsible for your own choices, actions, and results.

Legal Notice:

This book is copyright protected. This book is only for personal use. You cannot amend, distribute, sell, use, quote or paraphrase any part, of the content within this book, without the consent of the author or publisher.

Disclaimer Notice:

Please note the information contained within this document is for educational and entertainment purposes only. All effort has been expended to present accurate, up-to-date, and reliable, complete information. No warranties of any kind are declared or implied. Readers acknowledge that the author is not engaging in the rendering of legal, financial, medical or professional advice. The content within this book has been derived from various sources. Please consult a licensed professional before attempting any techniques outlined in this book.

By reading this document, the reader agrees that under no circumstances is the author responsible for any losses, direct or indirect, which are incurred as a result of the use of the information contained within this document, including, but not limited to, — errors, omissions, or inaccuracies.

Disclaimer: *I work as a health coach, but I'm not a doctor. The information provided in this book is solely intended for educational and informational purposes. It may not be the most suitable option for you or your specific circumstances. Please note that it should not be considered as medical advice or a substitute for professional medical advice, diagnosis, or treatment.*

CONTENTS

Introduction 5

1. GUT FEELINGS: THE SCIENCE BEHIND YOUR BODY'S SECOND BRAIN 9
   Your Gut Ecosystem: Balance and Diversity 10
   The Microbiome Revolution 11
   Gut-Brain Axis: The Fascinating Mind-Gut Connection 13
   Gut Health: Your Immune System's Secret Weapon! . 16
   Red Flags: Signs of Gut Imbalance 17
   The Science of Gut Health: Foundations and Facts . 19

2. FUEL YOUR GUT: THE POWER OF NUTRITION FOR A STRONGER YOU 21
   Plant-Based Power: Fiber for a Healthy Gut 23
   Anti-Inflammatory Foods 25
   Fabulous Fermented Foods: Natural (and Delicious!) Probiotic Sources 27
   Creating a Gut-Friendly Meal Plan 28
   Eating Your Way: Dietary Needs & Preferences 30

3. LIFESTYLE CHANGES FOR LASTING GUT HEALTH 33
   Sleep and Digestion: The Secret to a Restored Body 35
   Movement and Microbiota: Get Moving for Your Gut 37
   Mindful Eating: How Awareness Nourishes Your Gut 39
   Building a Happy Gut: Look Around You 40
   Stronger Together: How Community Boosts Your Health 42

4. OVERCOMING COMMON GUT HEALTH CHALLENGES 45
   Leaky Gut: Understanding and Healing 47
   Food Sensitivities and Allergies: Discovering What Works for You 48

The Role of Antibiotics and Gut Recovery	50
Gut Health in the Modern World: Balancing Wellness with Life's Demands	52
Trusting the Process: Overcoming Doubts on Your Gut Health Journey	54
5. CREATING YOUR UNIQUE GUT HEALTH PLAN	**58**
Setting Realistic Goals for Gut Health Transformation	59
Gut Health at Every Age: Adapting Practices for Every Life Stage	61
Perimenopause and the Gut-Hormone Connection	62
Integrating Gut Health with Other Wellness Goals	65
6. EXPANDING YOUR GUT HEALTH KNOWLEDGE	**68**
The Future of Gut Health: Breakthroughs and Innovations on the Horizon	70
Gut Health Myths and Misconceptions	72
The Role of Genetics in Gut Health	74
7. DELICIOUS & PRACTICAL: RECIPES TO BOOST YOUR GUT HEALTH	**77**
Lunchtime Solutions for Digestive Wellness	79
Dinners for a Happy Gut	81
Snack Smarter: Gut-Healthy Options	82
Refreshing Beverages for Gut Balance	84
Preparing Meals for Gut Health On-the-Go	85
Conclusion	89
Self Health Gut Guide BONUS QUESTIONS	93
References	113

INTRODUCTION

I wonder if you have ever felt like your body was trying to tell you something, but you couldn't quite figure out what it was saying? Well, that's how I felt for years as I struggled with a whole range of frustrating symptoms, from digestive issues and brain fog to a general sense of unwellness that I couldn't shake. It wasn't until I started investigating the fascinating world of gut health that I finally began to understand the root of my problems. And what a relief it was! This brings me to why I'm writing this book: I want others to feel the relief I have felt and get their life back, feeling healthy and happy once again. My own journey to wellness was so transformative that I was inspired to help others on their paths. This motivation led me to switch careers and complete training at the Institute for Integrative Nutrition. Now, as a Health Coach, I'm excited to share what I've learned with you.

But back to what I discovered. You see, our gut is so much more than what I thought it was: just a simple digestive system. It is in fact, a complex, interconnected network that plays a key role in our overall health and well-being. It's quite amazing to think that when our gut is out of balance, it can affect everything from our mental clarity to our energy levels and even our mood. It's a lot!

And unfortunately, (I'll get to the positive stuff soon, I promise!) despite the growing awareness of gut health, there's still a lot of confusion and misinformation out there. With so many conflicting dietary theories and overwhelming advice, it's easy to feel lost and unsure of where to start. That's why I wrote this book – to cut through all that noise and complication and provide a clear, accessible, practical guide to understanding and optimizing your gut health.

Self Health Gut Guide is certainly a book about digestion. But it's a holistic approach to wellness that recognizes the groundbreaking (yes, it's that big) connection between our gut and every other aspect of our lives. By looking into the latest scientific research and sharing practical, actionable, and easy tips, I aim to get you motivated and ready to take control of your health from the inside out.

Speaking of feeling motivated, I'd like you to, right now, take a moment to answer the questions below, which will guide you towards helping your *own* body. This is not a one-size-fits-all guidebook, so you'll need to be ready to tweak and adjust as needed.

Let's go!

What motivated you to start exploring gut health? Is there a specific goal you hope to achieve by improving your gut health? What is your current understanding of gut health? Are there any myths or misconceptions you realize you might have believed before?

First of all, well done! You've made the first step. Now, throughout these pages, we'll take a close look at the wonderful world of the gut microbiome and learn about how the trillions of bacteria that reside in our digestive tract influence our health in ways we never imagined. We'll look at the impact of your diet, your day-to-day stress levels, and the various lifestyle factors on our gut health, and find out some simple, effective strategies for promoting a thriving, diverse microbiome.

Sure, we'll get right into the science of gut health, but I want you to view this process as also an intensely personal journey, one that I've embarked on myself. As someone who has struggled with gut issues (I know, the struggle is real!) and worked my way around the often-confusing world of wellness, I understand the frustration and overwhelm that comes with trying to figure it all out. That's why I've made it my mission to create a resource for other sufferers that is not only informative, but I hope, also relatable and engaging.

I've designed each chapter of *Self Health Gut Guide* to build upon the last, gradually increasing your understanding of the gut-body connection and providing you with the tools you need to make lasting, meaningful changes. Along the way, you'll find reflective questions and prompts that are there to encourage you to apply what you're learning to your own life. At the end of the book, you'll have created an awesome, personalized roadmap for gut health and overall wellness that is bound to transform your life going forward. As a bonus, I included additional resources and questions for deeper self-discovery.

It doesn't matter if you're a complete beginner or a seasoned health enthusiast, I've written this book for you, keeping all levels in mind, and with the intention of meeting you wherever you are on your journey. We are all built differently, so I want you to feel guided and supported each step of the way as you explore the incredible potential of your own body.

Now, are you ready to transform your health from the inside out? To experience the energy, clarity, and vitality that comes with a thriving gut?! Then join me as we uncover the secrets of the gut-body connection and revel in just how powerful we are when we start listening to the wisdom within.

Let's get started, shall we?

1

GUT FEELINGS: THE SCIENCE BEHIND YOUR BODY'S SECOND BRAIN

Have you ever noticed how a bad meal can ruin your day (or keep you up at night with stomach pains), or how a stressful situation can leave your stomach in knots? It's no accident—our bodies are intricate systems, and at the heart of it all lies our gut. When you think about it, it makes total sense. I mean we've all heard, "You are what you eat." But somehow, we don't make the connection. I remember a time when I was stuck in a cycle of indigestion and fatigue, and no matter what I tried, I simply couldn't break free of it! It wasn't until I stumbled upon the fascinating world of gut health that I began to see a connection between what I ate, how I felt, and my overall vitality. This chapter is about exploring that connection. We'll study the incredible ecosystem living within us and how it plays a pivotal role in our overall wellness. Understanding this can transform not just how we eat, but how we live and feel every day.

YOUR GUT ECOSYSTEM: BALANCE AND DIVERSITY

Our gut is home to a vibrant little community of microorganisms, often referred to as the 'gut microbiome.' This ecosystem is a bustling metropolis of bacteria, both beneficial and pathogenic, living in a delicate balance. When this balance tips in favor of harmful bacteria, known as dysbiosis, it can lead to a cascade of health issues. Think of *homeostasis* as a seesaw, where beneficial bacteria keep the pathogenic ones in check. Achieving and maintaining this balance (keeping that seesaw from tipping over!) is essential for optimal gut function and our general health. A healthy gut supports digestion and nutrient absorption, and even influences our immune system.

Diversity within our gut microbiome is another key factor for maintaining health. A diverse microbiome acts like a beautiful, protective shield, boosting our resilience against infections and diseases. We can liken this to a garden with a variety of plants—each species contributes to the ecosystem's health, just like how a diverse microbiome supports ours. It really should be no surprise that studies have shown that people with a rich diversity of gut bacteria are less prone to illnesses, as these microorganisms play different roles in maintaining our health. They all have a special job to do and make up the most amazing team. On the other hand, it makes sense that monoculture diets, which rely heavily on a limited range of foods, can reduce this diversity, leaving us vulnerable to health problems.

There are no shortcuts to improving the diversity of your gut microbiome, like taking supplements or following strict diets. Instead, we need to welcome a lifestyle rich in variety and nutrients. And the bonus is that variety is the spice of life, right? More variety means more delicious foods to enjoy. But most importantly, incorporating a range of fiber-rich foods like fruits, vegetables, whole grains, and legumes can feed and nurture different bacterial species in your gut. Fermented foods, such as yogurt, kimchi, and sauerkraut, introduce beneficial bacteria and support a thriving microbial community. These dietary choices not only benefit your gut but also level up your health and vitality by promoting better digestion and improving your immune system.

To illustrate the far-reaching impact of microbial diversity, consider a study comparing the microbiomes of urban and rural populations. Researchers found that people living in rural areas, who typically consume a wider variety of unprocessed foods, have more diverse microbiomes compared to those in urban settings, where diets often include more processed foods. This diversity in rural populations has been linked to lower rates of allergies and autoimmune diseases. Impressive. Similarly, lifestyle changes can significantly alter microbiome composition. For instance, individuals who transition to plant-based diets often experience a positive shift in their gut flora, leading to noticeably improved health outcomes. These examples highlight the importance of working on building microbial diversity for a healthier life.

THE MICROBIOME REVOLUTION

Back to the bustling metropolis inside your body, teeming with life and activity. This is your gut microbiome, a collection of trillions of microorganisms, including bacteria, viruses, fungi, and protozoa, all living in your digestive tract. These tiny inhabitants play an integral role in your health, working symbiotically with your body. Bacteria are the most studied among them, often grabbing headlines for their role in digestion and nutrient absorption. But let's not overlook the others; viruses, fungi, and protozoa also contribute to maintaining this dynamic ecosystem. Each organism, much like a resident in a city works to help the community run smoothly. Each has its special role, and as you've learned already, together they help regulate digestion, support immune functions, and influence mood and cognition.

The study of the microbiome has a deep history, dating back to the early 20th century. However, it wasn't until recent advances in DNA sequencing technology that scientists could study this universe with precision. This technological leap has led to a welcome revolution in our understanding of how these microorganisms affect health. We now know that a well-balanced microbiome is key for maintaining homeostasis, which is the body's way of keeping a steady internal environment. We know that when this balance is disrupted, it can lead to a range of health issues, from metabolic diseases to mental health disorders.

I've said it before, and I'll say it again: the impact of the microbiome on health is huge. It aids in digesting food and extracting nutrients, processes that are vital for giving us the energy to live our lives well and to feel well in general.

But the role of the microbiome extends even further, to regulating metabolism and preventing conditions like obesity. By influencing how we store fat and control hunger hormones, the gut flora can significantly affect our weight and metabolic health. Furthermore, the microbiome's influence reaches the brain, affecting our mental health and mood regulation. This connection, often referred to as the *gut-brain axis*, shows just how much a healthy gut can lead to a healthy mind.

As you can imagine, several factors shape the composition of our microbiome, with diet being a primary influence. The foods we consume can either nourish beneficial bacteria or encourage the growth of pathogenic ones, and we've mentioned how diets rich in fiber and diverse nutrients support a thriving microbiome. In contrast, those loaded with processed foods and sugars can cause an imbalance. Antibiotics and medications, though sometimes necessary, can also disrupt the microbiome by wiping out beneficial bacteria, leaving room for harmful bacteria to thrive. Stress and sleep also play a critical role, as chronic stress and poor sleep can alter the microbiome, leading to imbalances that affect both physical and mental health.

Over to You! It's Time to Reflect...

Take a moment to reflect on your current diet and lifestyle. What small, sustainable changes are you willing to commit to in the short term as a starting point on your journey to better gut health? What changes can you make to introduce more diversity into your diet?

GUT-BRAIN AXIS: THE FASCINATING MIND-GUT CONNECTION

I bet you've felt butterflies in your stomach at some point in your life, perhaps before a big presentation. Or maybe you've had a gut-wrenching feeling during a stressful time or moment? This isn't just a coincidence—it's your gut and brain having a conversation; the gut-brain axis. This gut-brain axis is a complex communication system linking our gut and brain, signaling through pathways that include the vagus nerve, a sort of information superhighway.

The vagus nerve is a vital player here, transmitting messages between the gut and the brain at lightning speed. It's a two-way street, where the gut sends signals that can affect mood and cognition, while the brain sends signals that can alter gut function. You can see now where that churning stomach comes from! Our gut is also a neurotransmitter powerhouse, producing serotonin and dopamine, which are essential for mood regulation. This production means that our gut doesn't just digest the food we give it—it plays a massive role in our emotional and mental health.

The influence of gut health on mental well-being is significant. Studies have shown a strong correlation between gut health and mental health conditions like anxiety and depression. It's only becoming more well-known that an imbalance in gut bacteria, known as dysbiosis, can contribute to these conditions, signaling how deeply intertwined our mental and digestive systems are. For instance, people who have improved their gut health often report enhanced mental clarity and reduced anxiety symptoms. One very interesting case involved a group of individuals suffering from chronic depression. By focusing on restoring their gut health through diet and probiotics (more on that soon), many experienced a noticeable improvement in mood and mental clarity, highlighting the gut's impact on the mind. It's time to rethink mental health and focus on improving our bodies, not just our minds or mindset.

Let's talk a bit more about diet in nurturing this mind-gut connection. Omega-3 fatty acids, found in fish and flaxseeds, are known to support both brain and gut health, boosting cognitive function and emotional balance. Antioxidants and polyphenols, found in colorful fruits and vegetables, act like a wonderful shield, protecting your cells from damage and supporting immune health. These compounds have been shown to promote the growth of beneficial gut bacteria, which in turn enhance your body's natural defenses. Zinc and vitamin D are equally vital, acting as the backbone of a resilient immune system. Zinc helps maintain the integrity of your gut lining, while vitamin D modulates immune responses, ensuring they are neither too weak nor overly aggressive.

We all know that sugar and processed foods are not good for us, but reducing them can have a similar effect, helping to clear the mental fog that many of us experience—something to think about when reaching for too many chocolates or sweet treats.

The good news (I told you I'd be sharing some!) is that these small, and relatively easy dietary changes can act like a reset button for your brain, bringing forth a clearer, more focused mind. Isn't that what we all want, to feel more alert and emotionally balanced? And to think it only takes a few tweaks to your diet. I'm not here to tell you to avoid junk food. I just want to share with you the effects of different foods on your body so that you can improve your health. And I know, this doesn't happen overnight, it's a step-by-step process, so go easy on yourself as you make those steps.

Recent research into the gut-brain axis has opened up some other exciting possibilities. Scientists are looking into new therapies that target this connection, potentially offering new treatments for neurological disorders. These therapies focus on restoring balance in the microbiome to improve mental health outcomes. The implications are vast, suggesting that by caring for our gut, we might also be safeguarding our brain health. For example, the prospect of using gut health to address conditions like Parkinson's or depression is more than promising. This burgeoning field of study is shedding light on how we can use our diet to fuel our bodies *and support* our mental health.

The gut-brain axis shows just how interconnected our intelligent bodies truly are; a reminder that when we nourish one part, we nourish the whole. Grasping and incorporating this connection can transform our approach to health, blending nutrition and mindfulness into our daily lives.

GUT HEALTH: YOUR IMMUNE SYSTEM'S SECRET WEAPON!

At the heart of the busy community that is your gut, lies the gut-associated lymphoid tissue (GALT), which is really the unsung hero of your immune system. This tissue acts as a vigilant sentinel, tirelessly working to differentiate between friend and foe. When your gut microbiome is in harmony, GALT can effectively regulate immune responses so that your body isn't on high alert unnecessarily. Essentially, GALT coordinates a dynamic dance between your gut microbiota and immune cells, guiding your body's natural defenses. When beneficial bacteria flourish, they help train immune cells to recognize harmful pathogens, reducing the risk of chronic inflammation and autoimmune disorders.

As we've learned, when this balance is disrupted, poor gut health can weaken your body's defenses, making you more susceptible to infections and inflammation. Chronic inflammation is a silent saboteur, quietly wreaking havoc on your health while you go about your day. Yet, a healthy gut can be your greatest ally in reducing this inflammation. And so, we need to nurture a robust microbiome so that you can boost your immune resilience, potentially even influencing how effectively vaccines work. You see, vaccines rely on a well-functioning immune system to teach your body how to fight off future infections. Evidence suggests that a healthy gut can enhance this process, leading to better immune responses and protection from diseases. This is pretty powerful stuff!

Research continues to uncover fascinating insights into the gut-immune connection. For instance, as mentioned briefly earlier, studies have demonstrated the immune-modulating effects of *probiotics*, which are live bacteria that bestow great health benefits when consumed in adequate amounts. Probiotics can enhance your gut microbiome, promoting a balanced immune response and reducing inflammation. They may even help prevent or alleviate symptoms of conditions like irritable bowel syndrome and inflammatory bowel diseases. Looking ahead, researchers are exploring new ways to leverage this connection, potentially creating innovative treatments that use the power of the microbiome to support immune health.

Then there's the well-publicized study that found that a high-fiber diet can alter the composition of the gut microbiota, promoting the growth of beneficial bacteria and reducing inflammation.

RED FLAGS: SIGNS OF GUT IMBALANCE

It's surprising how often we overlook the subtle messages our body sends us. For example, we might brush off persistent bloating or occasional gas or irregular bowel movements as just a part of life, but these symptoms often act as the body's red flags, signaling to us that something deeper is going on. You can think of these signs perhaps as being like the flashing check engine light on your car's dashboard. If left unchecked, these discomforts can cascade into more severe issues. Beyond the digestive system, an imbalanced gut can manifest as unexplained fatigue, the kind that lingers no matter how much you rest. Skin issues, too, often trace back to gut health, with acne or eczema reflecting internal inflammation.

The gut lining, when healthy, acts as a necessary barrier, selectively allowing welcome nutrients to pass while keeping nasty toxins out. But when this lining becomes permeable—a condition often referred to as "leaky gut"—it can lead to systemic inflammation. This inflammation affects the gut, but can also spread, influencing everything from energy levels to skin health. Understanding these connections allows you to take the necessary steps to heal from within.

So, how do you evaluate whether your gut is in balance? One of the most straightforward methods is maintaining a *food and symptom diary*. Simply track what you eat and how you feel afterward. Over time, patterns will emerge, revealing food triggers and times when symptoms flare up. Additionally, over-the-counter gut health tests can provide insights into your microbiome's state. These tests, though not a replacement for professional advice, can offer a snapshot of your gut flora, highlighting areas of concern.

It's important to note here though, that it's one thing to discover you have some issues with your gut health, and it's another to recognize when to seek professional help. So, if persistent symptoms linger despite lifestyle changes, or if you experience severe digestive disorders and significant pain/discomfort/it limits your daily life, it's time to consult a healthcare provider. Ignoring these signs can lead to more significant health issues down the road. There's no need to suffer endlessly! Healthcare professionals can offer diagnostics to find out exactly what's going on and provide tailored advice to restore balance and health to get you back on track. This way, you're not just treating symptoms; you're addressing the root cause.

Over to You! It's Time to Reflect...

Consider keeping a journal to track your dietary choices and any changes you make. Reflect on how these adjustments affect your overall well-being, noting improvements or setbacks.

THE SCIENCE OF GUT HEALTH: FOUNDATIONS AND FACTS

The human digestive system really is a masterpiece of natural engineering! Take a moment to think about its complex network of organs, all working in harmony to transform the food you eat into the energy that fuels our every move. It starts at the mouth and winds its way through the esophagus, stomach, and intestines, finally ending at the rectum. Each section plays a distinct role in breaking down nutrients and absorbing them into our bloodstream. And then, beyond the mere mechanics of digestion, our gut is teeming with life—those trillions of microorganisms.

Despite the growing body of evidence, misconceptions about gut health persist. One common myth is that all bacteria are harmful and should be avoided. In reality, while some bacteria can cause disease, many are beneficial and play key roles in maintaining our health. Another misconception is that gut health is irrelevant to mental health. Yet, research has consistently shown that the gut-brain connection is real, with our gut microbiota impacting our mood and cognitive function, energy levels, and overall well-being.

Looking ahead, the future of gut health science is filled with exciting possibilities. For example, advances in *personalized nutrition and microbiome profiling* are paving the way for tailored health recommendations. In the not-too-distant future, you could imagine receiving a diet plan specifically designed to optimize your unique microbiome, improving your physical and mental health in ways previously unimaginable. Additionally, the development of *microbiome therapeutics*—medicines or interventions that target the microbiome—holds promise for treating various conditions, from obesity to mental health disorders. These innovations could completely revolutionize how we approach health and medicine, shifting the focus from treating symptoms to addressing underlying causes.

2

FUEL YOUR GUT: THE POWER OF NUTRITION FOR A STRONGER YOU

Let's take a closer look at your gut microbiota. It's fueled by two essential players—*probiotics* and *prebiotics*. It can be handy to think of them as the gardeners of your internal ecosystem. Probiotics are the live bacteria that we often hear touted as "good bacteria." They are the friendly tenants that help maintain harmony in your gut, playing an essential role in digestion and immunity. On the other hand, prebiotics are the indigestible fibers that act as nourishment for these bacteria, encouraging them to grow and flourish. They're an awesome team, and together, they create a balanced, thriving environment that impacts your health in big ways.

Now, you might be wondering where to find these beneficial components. Let's start with probiotics. They're abundant in fermented foods like yogurt and kefir. These foods are not just tasty but also brimming with live cultures that can replenish your gut's bacterial population. When you enjoy a serving of yogurt, you're essentially introducing billions of helpful bacteria into your digestive system! And it's so easy! Kefir, a tangy, fermented milk drink, offers similar benefits, often with an even more diverse range of probiotic strains. These foods provide a delicious and natural way to boost your gut health.

Prebiotics, on the other hand, are found in fiber-rich foods like bananas, onions, and garlic. They are pretty amazing at quietly feeding the good bacteria and helping them to thrive. While you may not notice their effects immediately, they work behind the scenes to improve digestion and nutrient absorption. Bananas are a convenient snack that not only satisfies hunger but also supports your gut. Onions and garlic, often used as flavor enhancers in cooking, pack a powerful prebiotic punch, making them a staple in any gut-friendly kitchen.

Including these elements in your diet can lead to a cascade of health benefits. With a well-fed gut microbiota, you'll likely experience improved digestion and more efficient nutrient absorption. This means less bloating and better energy levels, as your body can better extract and utilize the nutrients from the food you eat. And as you know already, a balanced gut flora can enhance your immune system. A study from the Mayo Clinic highlights how probiotics and prebiotics work together to support this healthy balance, emphasizing their role in maintaining a healthy microbiome and preventing digestive issues.

To make the most of these benefits, consider some guidelines for consuming probiotics and prebiotics. Aim to include a serving of probiotic-rich food, like yogurt or kefir, in your daily meals. When selecting probiotic supplements, look for products that contain *multiple strains* and a *high CFU (colony-forming unit)* count, as these indicate the presence of live and active cultures. For prebiotics, focus on incorporating a variety of fiber-rich foods into your diet. This can be as simple as adding a banana to your breakfast or tossing onions and garlic into your stir-fry. These small changes can have a significant impact on your gut health.

Over to You! It's Time to Reflect...

Take a few minutes to assess your current diet. How often do you include probiotic and prebiotic foods in your meals? Consider keeping a food diary for a week to track your intake. Note any changes in your digestion or overall well-being as you increase these gut-friendly foods. Reflect on how these dietary adjustments affect your energy levels and mood.

PLANT-BASED POWER: FIBER FOR A HEALTHY GUT

Your digestive system is like a well-oiled machine, one that relies heavily on a key component—dietary fiber. This often-overlooked nutrient is indispensable for maintaining a healthy gut environment. Fiber works its magic by promoting bowel regularity, acting like a kind of natural broom that sweeps through your intestines, ensuring everything runs smoothly! It keeps things moving at a steady pace, too, preventing the discomfort of constipation and irregular bowel movements. You feel well when your digestion is regular, but it means that you're also optimizing how efficiently your body absorbs nutrients. As you're beginning to understand, this efficiency can have a ripple effect on your energy levels and overall well-being.

Now, let's talk about the different types of fiber, each serving a unique purpose. *Soluble fiber* dissolves in water to form a gel-like substance, which helps lower cholesterol and stabilize blood sugar levels. It's the kind of fiber that makes oats such a heart-healthy breakfast choice.

On the other hand, *insoluble fiber* doesn't dissolve in water. Instead, it adds bulk to your stool, which helps food pass more quickly through the stomach and intestines, giving you those regular bowel movements.

To reap the benefits of both types of fiber, adding a variety of high-fiber foods to your diet is key. Lentils, beans, and whole grains like quinoa and brown rice are excellent sources. These foods not only provide fiber but also pack a punch of protein and essential nutrients. Fruits, too, offer a delicious way to boost your fiber intake. Apples, with their crisp texture and sweet taste, are perfect for an on-the-go snack. Berries, like strawberries and blueberries, are rich in antioxidants and provide a generous dose of fiber.

Increasing your fiber intake might seem daunting at first, but it's really quite simple. Start by gradually adding fiber-rich foods to your diet to give your digestive system time to adjust. Consider topping your morning cereal or yogurt with chia seeds, a small but mighty source of fiber and omega-3 fatty acids. Flaxseeds are another excellent addition, easily sprinkled over salads or blended into smoothies. These small seeds pack a powerful fiber punch, boosting your gut health without much effort. Experimenting with fiber-rich recipes can also make this process enjoyable. Try a hearty lentil soup or a colorful grain bowl filled with a variety of vegetables and legumes.

Over to You! It's Time to Reflect...

Recipe Challenge

Challenge yourself to create a new fiber-rich recipe. Start by choosing a base like quinoa or lentils and add a mix of colorful vegetables and your favorite spices. Share your creation with friends or family and notice how including more fiber can be both delicious and beneficial for your gut health.

As you gradually increase your fiber intake, remember to *stay hydrated*. Fiber works best with adequate water, helping it move smoothly through your digestive tract. If you're used to a lower-fiber diet, increasing fiber too quickly can lead to bloating or gas. But don't worry—these symptoms usually subside as your body adjusts.

ANTI-INFLAMMATORY FOODS

While a healthy gut is busy and happy, inflammation acts a bit like traffic congestion, slowing everything down and creating chaos. Chronic inflammation irritates your gut, but it can also disrupt its function, leading to a range of digestive disorders, such as a "leaky gut," which we described earlier. The constant stress on your gut can spiral into more serious issues like irritable bowel syndrome or inflammatory bowel disease, making the management of inflammation crucial.

The good news is that certain foods have natural anti-inflammatory properties that can help soothe your gut's turmoil. Turmeric and ginger are two such powerhouses. While they add delicious flavors to our dishes, they also contain compounds like curcumin and gingerol, which have been shown to reduce inflammation and support gut health. Including them in your daily diet can be as simple as sprinkling turmeric on your morning eggs or adding ginger to your tea!

Then there's fatty fish, such as salmon and mackerel, which are rich in omega-3 fatty acids, which are well-known for their anti-inflammatory effects. These acids can help reduce the production of inflammatory molecules, providing a protective effect on your gut.

Consider starting your day with a turmeric-infused smoothie—just blend some turmeric with your favorite fruits, a bit of ginger, and a splash of almond milk for a delicious and gut-friendly breakfast. When cooking, swap out refined oils for olive oil, which is rich in monounsaturated fats and polyphenols that can help reduce inflammation.

Adding these foods can make a big difference over time. When you incorporate more anti-inflammatory foods into your diet, you'll likely notice not just improvements in gut health, but also a boost in how you feel every day.

What's exciting is that the benefits of an anti-inflammatory diet extend beyond gut health. You may find that joint pain and arthritis symptoms are reduced, thanks to the body's decreased inflammatory response. This diet is also linked to a lower risk of chronic diseases such as heart disease and type 2 diabetes. When your body is less inflamed, it's more efficient at repairing and maintaining itself, which can lead to improved energy levels and a greater sense of vitality. This is because, with inflammation under control, your body is able to focus on functioning optimally, allowing you to enjoy life more fully.

Keep in mind here that what works for one person might not work for another. Try different foods and recipes to find what makes your body feel its best! And remember, it's okay to ask for help if you're unsure where to start. Consulting with a nutritionist or dietitian can provide personalized guidance tailored to your needs. Stay curious and open-minded as you experiment and always celebrate your progress, no matter how small it may seem. What's most important here is that you are taking active steps to improve your health, and you should feel proud of that!

FABULOUS FERMENTED FOODS: NATURAL (AND DELICIOUS!) PROBIOTIC SOURCES

Think for a moment about a process where simple sugars are transformed into tangy, complex flavors, enhancing both taste and nutrition. This is the magic of fermentation, a natural process where microorganisms like bacteria convert sugars into acids or alcohol. It's a time-honored method that has been a part of the human diet for centuries, and many have used it to preserve food and enjoy its health benefits. This process creates an environment rich in probiotics, the live bacteria that support gut health. When foods ferment, they develop a higher content of these beneficial bacteria, turning ordinary ingredients into gut-friendly superfoods.

Let's check out some of the fermented foods that can easily find a place in your kitchen. Kimchi, a staple in Korean cuisine, combines cabbage and radishes with spices to create a spicy, flavorful dish that can enliven any meal. Sauerkraut, its milder cousin, offers a crunchier texture and a tangy taste that's perfect for sandwiches or salads. Miso, a fermented soybean paste, is a versatile ingredient that can be used in soups, dressings, or marinades. These foods are not only delicious but also readily available in most grocery stores, making them accessible additions to your diet. Each serves as a natural source of probiotics, supporting your digestive health while adding depth and flavor to your meals.

So, fermentation introduces probiotics, but what many don't know is that it also enhances the bioavailability of nutrients, making them easier for your body to absorb. They basically unleash the full potential of the food you eat! When nutrients become more accessible, your body can use them more effectively, which means it's a win-win for your taste buds and your health.

Integrating these foods into your daily routine really is very easy. Start small by adding a spoonful of sauerkraut to your sandwich or salad. Its tangy flavor complements a variety of dishes, providing a probiotic boost with minimal effort. Miso can be a versatile addition to your cooking arsenal. Try using it as a base for a comforting soup by mixing it with hot water and your choice of vegetables and proteins. This simple dish not only warms you up but also supports your gut health. If you're feeling adventurous, experiment with kimchi. Its spicy kick pairs well with rice bowls, tacos, or even as a topping for a homemade pizza.

The beauty of fermented foods lies in their adaptability. You don't need to overhaul your entire diet to enjoy its benefits. Instead, think of them as enhancements, small additions that can make a big difference. As you experiment with these foods, you'll likely find new favorites that keep your taste buds happy and your gut thriving!

CREATING A GUT-FRIENDLY MEAL PLAN

Creating a meal plan that supports your gut health is all about welcoming a bit more diversity in your food choices so that you are getting a well-rounded intake of nutrients. Vegetables, fruits, whole grains, lean proteins, and healthy fats each play vital roles in nourishing your gut. A diverse selection of foods provides a wide array of vitamins, minerals, and fibers that are crucial for maintaining a balanced microbiome. Eating a variety of food groups supports your digestive system but also means your body gets a broad spectrum of nutrients, which is excellent for your health and energy levels.

To maintain this balance, meal planning is your best friend. Start by preparing a weekly shopping list. This list should reflect a variety of fresh produce, whole grains, proteins, and healthy fats, and don't forget fermented foods and foods packed with probiotics. Planning ahead means you won't forget to eat better, and also helps you avoid impulsive choices that may not support your gut health.

Consider dedicating a day to batch cooking, where you can prepare multiple meals at once. This approach saves time during the week and ensures you have healthy options readily available as opposed to feeling tired and eating something unhealthy. We've all been there! Portion meals into containers, so you can grab them quickly, because if it's too hard to access, you'll weaken and go for an easier option. This method supports your gut and helps you stick to your health goals.

For breakfast, consider starting your day with overnight oats topped with chia seeds and berries. Not only is this meal easy to prepare, but it also offers a rich supply of fiber and antioxidants to kickstart your metabolism. As you move into lunch, a quinoa salad with mixed vegetables and a refreshing lemon dressing can provide a satisfying midday meal. Quinoa, being a complete protein, offers all nine essential amino acids, while the vegetables add color, flavor, and nutrients that support your gut's ecosystem. Perfect! These meals need to be delicious, but they're also designed to keep you feeling full and energized throughout the day without causing a mid-afternoon slump.

The beauty of a well-crafted meal plan lies in its adaptability to your unique dietary preferences. Whether you're vegetarian, gluten-free, or following any specific dietary guidelines, you can tailor your meals accordingly. For instance, swap animal proteins for plant-based options like lentils or chickpeas, which are high in protein and fiber. For those avoiding gluten, whole grains like quinoa and rice are excellent substitutes that provide similar benefits without gluten. The key is flexibility and planning.

Feel proud of yourself, you're creating habits that promote a healthier lifestyle, one meal at a time.

EATING YOUR WAY: DIETARY NEEDS & PREFERENCES

Working your way through dietary restrictions can feel overwhelming at first. You might be gluten-free, dairy-free, or following a low-FODMAP diet. Whatever it is, these limitations don't have to be barriers. With an abundance of alternatives, you can still enjoy meals that support a healthy gut. For those avoiding gluten, products made with almond flour or coconut flour are excellent substitutes, offering both texture and flavor without the gluten. Almond flour, in particular, is a favorite for baking, lending a nutty richness to gluten-free banana bread, turning it from a dietary necessity into a delightful treat. If dairy is off the table, look into dairy-free yogurt alternatives made from coconut milk or almond milk. These options provide the creamy consistency we love, along with a wealth of nutrients that keep your gut happy.

This stage is all about understanding your body's unique needs and finding what works best for you. Consulting with a nutritionist or dietitian can provide invaluable guidance, helping you tailor your diet to meet both your health goals and dietary restrictions.

These professionals can offer personalized advice, suggest delicious alternative foods, and help you understand complicated labels, all the while making sure you get the nutrients you need without triggering any adverse reactions. Their expertise can demystify dietary restrictions, turning a potential challenge into an opportunity for trying something new.

Adapting recipes to fit your dietary needs certainly doesn't mean compromising on flavor or enjoyment. Simple substitutions can transform traditional recipes into gut-friendly versions that cater to your specific needs. For example, gluten-free banana bread using almond flour not only meets gluten-free requirements but also offers a deliciously moist and flavorful alternative to its wheat-based counterpart. Similarly, dairy-free yogurt made with coconut milk provides a creamy, satisfying base for parfaits or smoothies, without the lactose. These adaptable recipes allow you to enjoy the foods you love while supporting your gut health, proving that dietary restrictions are merely guidelines, not limitations.

Dining out can present its own set of challenges, but with a bit of preparation, you can maintain your gut health while enjoying meals outside your home. When choosing a restaurant, look for those with diverse menu options that can accommodate various dietary needs. Many establishments are now more aware of dietary restrictions and offer gluten-free, dairy-free, and other options clearly marked on their menus. When ordering, don't hesitate to ask about cooking methods and ingredients. Knowing whether a dish contains hidden gluten or dairy can help you make informed choices. Most chefs these days are used to requests and are happy to accommodate you, by perhaps swapping out an ingredient or preparing a dish in a specific way.

I want you to know here that things have changed. These strategies are no longer about surviving dietary restrictions but thriving within them. When you understand your needs and have checked out alternatives, you can turn what seems like a limitation into a source of strength. With a positive mindset, you can focus on the possibilities rather than the restrictions. And besides, a little creativity in the kitchen can be fun!

The next chapter will further expand on lifestyle changes that complement your dietary efforts, helping you create a holistic approach to gut health.

3
LIFESTYLE CHANGES FOR LASTING GUT HEALTH

Can you think of a moment when stress crept into your life uninvited? Maybe it happens often for you, or perhaps it's only when something out of the ordinary that makes you comfortable happens, like the morning of a big presentation, or the day when your to-do list seemed longer than the hours in the day, and you felt stressed and overwhelmed. I bet you felt that tightening in your stomach, the churn of unease, as if your gut itself was reacting to the chaos in your mind. It's more than just a feeling—it's actually your body's stress response in action, organized by a complex system known as the hypothalamic-pituitary-adrenal (HPA) axis. Yes, it really is a thing! This axis coordinates the release of cortisol, that hormone that prepares your body to handle stress. While critical, it is crucial for managing short-term stress; when levels remain elevated due to chronic or intense stress, it can wreak havoc on your gut health.

The impact of cortisol on your gut is multifaceted. High cortisol levels can increase gut permeability (the "leaky gut"), where the gut lining becomes more porous. This allows unwanted substances to pass into the bloodstream, potentially leading to inflammation and digestive disorders like irritable bowel syndrome (IBS) or inflammatory bowel disease (IBD). The balance of your gut microbiota can also be disrupted, leading to dysbiosis, which may manifest as bloating, abdominal pain, and irregular bowel movements. Stress can really throw a wrench into the finely tuned machine of your digestive system, causing it to misfire in ways that affect your overall health.

Recognizing the symptoms of stress-related gut issues is the first step in regaining control. You might notice abdominal pain, a sense of bloating, or changes in your bowel habits, such as diarrhea or constipation, during or after stressful periods. These symptoms are your body's way of signaling that it's time to hit the brakes and address the underlying stressors. If you continue to ignore them, eventually, something's going to give. But fear not, because there are easy, practical things you can do to manage stress and its impact on your gut health.

One of the simplest yet most effective ways to combat stress is through deep breathing exercises. Taking slow, intentional breaths can activate your parasympathetic nervous system, which helps counteract the stress response and promote a sense of calm. You can think of your breath as a gentle wave washing over you, soothing tension, calming your gut, and bringing clarity. Adding yoga and meditation to your daily routine can further enhance this effect. These practices encourage mindfulness, relaxation, and deep breathing, providing a sanctuary from the rush and stress of daily life. By dedicating even a few minutes each day to these activities, you can create a buffer against stress that protects both your mind and your gut.

Building resilience against stress should also include strengthening your ability to handle stress over the long term. Establishing a consistent daily routine can anchor you amidst life's uncertainties, offering a sense of predictability and stability. Simple changes can make a big difference! You might like to start your day with a calming cup of herbal tea (soaking up the moment rather than scrolling on your phone), take a walk after lunch, do yoga and meditation, or wind down with a book before bed. All of these simple rituals create touchpoints of calm throughout your day. Prioritizing self-care and relaxation activities is equally important. Make time for the things that bring you joy, such as painting, gardening, or spending time with loved ones. These activities fill up your emotional reserves, making you more resilient in the face of stress. This holistic approach recognizes that your gut is truly a partner toward lasting health and vitality.

Over to You! It's Time to Reflect...

Carve out a moment to reflect on your current stress management practices. What are the stressors in your life that most affect your gut health? Consider keeping a journal to track these stressors and your body's response. Identify at least one new stress-reducing activity you can add to your routine, such as a breathing exercise, a yoga session, or a short mindfulness meditation. Reflect on how these changes impact both your stress levels and your gut health over the coming weeks.

SLEEP AND DIGESTION: THE SECRET TO A RESTORED BODY

Ever woken up after a restless night, feeling more than just groggy? Perhaps your stomach's not quite right, maybe even a bit upset. That's no coincidence. Your sleep and gut health are more intertwined than you might think. At the heart of this connection is your circadian rhythm, the body's internal clock that regulates sleep-wake cycles and impacts various bodily functions, including digestion. What many of us don't know, or forget, is that when you sleep well, your circadian rhythm helps synchronize the release of digestive enzymes and hormones, promoting efficient digestion. But when sleep is disrupted, this rhythm is thrown off, leading to chaos in your gut.

So, sleep deprivation doesn't just make us tired; it actually alters the composition of our gut microbiota. Studies have shown that a lack of sleep can lead to an unfavorable shift in gut bacteria, which may increase the risk of gastrointestinal disorders. Poor sleep can also slow down digestion, leading to issues like acid reflux, bloating, and irregular bowel movements. The longer this cycle continues, the more it can impact your gut health, creating a feedback loop that's hard to break. Rest and recovery are what your mind, body, and gut need.

Start by working on your sleep hygiene by setting a regular sleep schedule, going to bed, and waking up at the same time every day, even on weekends. This consistency reinforces your body's natural rhythms, making it easier to fall asleep and stay asleep. While it sounds obvious, creating a restful sleep environment is equally important. Keep your bedroom cool, dark, and quiet, and while I know it's challenging, banish screens at least an hour before bed. The blue light emitted by phones, tablets, and computers really does interfere with the production of melatonin, the hormone that signals your body it's time to sleep. Instead, try unwinding with a book or some gentle stretching exercises, or yoga to prepare your body for rest.

Consider the experiences of individuals who've seen significant improvements in their gut health through better sleep practices.

Take Jenna, for instance, who struggled with persistent IBS symptoms for years. After committing to a stricter sleep schedule and making her bedroom a sanctuary for rest, she noticed a marked reduction in her symptoms. Her bloating decreased, and her bowel movements became more regular, leading to a newfound sense of comfort and control over her body. Or think about Eric, who found that cutting out late-night screen time and incorporating a pre-sleep meditation routine helped him fall asleep faster and wake up feeling refreshed. His improved sleep quality translated to fewer digestive issues, too, reinforcing the powerful connection between rest and gut health.

By prioritizing quality sleep, you're giving your gut the best chance to function optimally.

Note: If you are still having trouble sleeping, consult with a professional who can help provide you with some natural support.

MOVEMENT AND MICROBIOTA: GET MOVING FOR YOUR GUT

Have you ever noticed how a brisk walk can clear your mind or how a good workout leaves you feeling refreshed and invigorated? There's a reason for that. It's well-known that exercise benefits our muscles and heart, but it also helps, you guessed it...maintain a healthy gut. This is because physical activity boosts gut microbial diversity. And as we know, this diversity is important because a varied microbiome is more resilient and better equipped to fend off disease.

However, not all exercises are created equal when it comes to gut health. Aerobic activities such as walking, cycling, or swimming are excellent choices. They increase your heart rate and promote circulation, which helps oxygenate the body's tissues, including the gut! These activities also boost the production of short-chain fatty acids, beneficial compounds that nourish the cells lining your intestines. Strength training, too, can play a vital role. By building muscle, you help regulate blood sugar levels and improve metabolism, both of which are beneficial for maintaining a healthy gut. The combination of aerobic and strength training exercises creates a holistic approach to wellness, supporting not just your gut but your entire body.

When you're starting an exercise routine, it's essential to set realistic and achievable fitness goals. Begin by assessing your current fitness level and consider what you enjoy doing. Setting goals that are attainable yet challenging can keep you motivated and engaged. Whether it's walking for thirty minutes a day, cycling a few times a week, lifting weights at the gym, or joining a yoga class, consistency is key. Try balancing different types of exercises to create a well-rounded routine. Pairing aerobic activities with strength training can yield the best results, providing comprehensive benefits for your gut and overall health.

Adding movement to your daily life doesn't have to be a chore. There are plenty of simple ways to stay active without drastically changing your routine. Taking the stairs instead of the elevator is a small but effective way to increase your daily activity level. Consider parking further from your destination to add extra steps to your day. During work breaks, take short walks around the office or outside if possible. These brief moments of movement can really add up, contributing to your daily exercise goals and supporting your gut health.

You can also find joy in movement and integrate it into your everyday life by being aware of chances to move. You could dance around your living room, play a game of tag with your kids, take a leisurely bike ride through the park, or even ride to work. The goal is to keep your body moving in ways that feel good and fit into your lifestyle. And naturally, the more you enjoy the activities you choose, the more likely you are to stick with them.

MINDFUL EATING: HOW AWARENESS NOURISHES YOUR GUT

How long has it been since you sat down for a meal, truly savored each bite, and been fully present in the moment? This is the essence of *mindful eating*, a practice that encourages you to focus on the sensory experience of eating. When we eat mindfully, we slow down in order to notice the colors, textures, and flavors of our food, as well as the sounds it makes as we chew. By homing in on these details, we create a deeper connection with what we're eating. We enjoy our food more when we eat mindfully as we savor all of the flavors and textures, but eating this way can also lead to a reduction in overeating and digestive stress. When you eat mindfully, you're more likely to recognize your body's hunger and fullness cues, too, helping you avoid the discomfort that comes from eating too much or too quickly. This simple awareness can actually transform your relationship with food, turning meals into nourishing and enjoyable experiences rather than simply eating because you're hungry, or even worse, eating on the run.

To become more mindful during meals, start by slowing down. Chew each bite thoroughly and savor the flavors as they unfold. This can also lead to reduced bloating, as your body has the time it needs to process food properly. Many people find that when they eat mindfully, they feel more satisfied with smaller portions, as they are more in tune with their body's hunger cues. Pay attention to your body's signals and try eating without distractions like

TV or smartphones so that you can more easily listen to your body's needs and respond accordingly, not to mention feel more grateful for the food you are eating. By focusing on the act of eating, you become more attuned to how different foods affect your body, making it easier to choose meals that make you feel good long after the last bite. This simple shift in how you approach eating can have some significant effects on your digestion and overall satisfaction with meals.

One exercise to practice mindful eating is the famous raisin exercise. It involves taking a single raisin and examining it closely, noting its texture, color, and smell. As you place it in your mouth, focus on the sensations it creates, chewing slowly and intentionally. This simple practice can be eye-opening, teaching you to appreciate the subtleties of flavor and texture that you might otherwise overlook, and helping you apply what you've learned when eating other foods.

Over to You! It's Time to Reflect...

After eating, take a few minutes to jot down how you feel, both physically and emotionally, after eating. Reflect on what you enjoyed about the meal and how it affected your body. This practice can help you identify patterns and preferences, guiding you toward food choices that support your health and well-being.

BUILDING A HAPPY GUT: LOOK AROUND YOU

It might surprise you to learn that the environment you live and work in can significantly affect your gut health. Pollutants and allergens are often the invisible culprits that disrupt our internal harmony. These can come from everyday sources like household cleaning products, air fresheners, or even the materials of furniture and flooring. Each of these elements has the potential to affect the delicate balance of your gut microbiota, leading to inflammation and digestive discomfort.

Reducing your exposure to environmental toxins is another practical step you can take to support your gut health. You can start by choosing natural cleaning products that avoid harsh chemicals. Many of these products are just as effective as their chemical-laden counterparts but without the potential negative impacts on your health. Consider swapping out plastic food storage containers for glass or stainless-steel options. Plastics can leach harmful chemicals into your food, especially when heated, contributing to toxicity in the body over time. Even small changes in how you store and prepare food can make a noticeable difference in reducing your overall toxin load.

Optimizing your home environment for gut health means taking a little extra time to create a space that supports not just your body, but your mind and spirit as well. Things like introducing houseplants into your living space can be a simple and effective way to purify the air. Plants like the Peace Lily or Snake Plant are known for their ability to filter toxins and improve air quality, which benefits your respiratory health and, indirectly, your gut. Pretty amazing, right?

Making sure your home has adequate ventilation is another key factor, as it helps to circulate fresh air and remove indoor pollutants. Open windows often, use fans to promote airflow, and consider investing in a good quality air purifier if needed. These changes can totally transform your home into a haven of health.

To illustrate the impact of these environmental changes, I want to share with you the experiences of individuals who have taken steps to detoxify their living spaces. Take Emily, who suffered from chronic bloating and fatigue. By switching to natural cleaning products and adding houseplants to her home, she noticed a marked improvement in her symptoms. Her energy levels increased, and she found herself feeling more vibrant and healthier.

Similarly, Niko, who dealt with frequent headaches and digestive issues, took action by reducing his use of plastic and ensuring his home was well-ventilated. Over time, he experienced fewer headaches and a significant reduction in digestive discomfort. These stories highlight the transformative potential of creating a gut-friendly environment.

By making mindful choices about the products you use and the spaces you inhabit, you can create an environment that supports your gut and general health and happiness.

STRONGER TOGETHER: HOW COMMUNITY BOOSTS YOUR HEALTH

I'd like you, for a moment, to think about a time when you felt truly connected to someone. Maybe it was sharing a joke with a close friend or confiding in a family member. While these moments sure are heartwarming and help us feel connected and heard, they're also vital to our health. And that includes the well-being of our gut because having strong social connections can reduce stress significantly, which, as we've seen, has a significant impact on gut health. When you're surrounded by supportive relationships, your body feels it too, often translating into fewer digestive woes. Even better for your health than lovely social connections is *shared health journeys* with others. Exercising or making health changes together can be very motivating and help you to stick to your wellness goals. What could be better than thriving mentally, socially, and physically?

You could catch up with a friend and keep each other accountable for joint walks or exercise goals, or you could build a supportive community around yourself. Start by looking for local wellness groups or classes that align with your interests. There are plenty of activities that can enhance social bonds while also promoting gut health. It could be a yoga class at a nearby studio or a cooking workshop focused on healthy meals. Hosting a healthy potluck dinner is a fantastic way to bring people together and share nutritious meals. Invite friends or family to each contribute a dish, focusing on recipes that are both delicious and gut-friendly. This not only allows you to enjoy a variety of foods but also opens up like-minded conversations about health and wellness.

Another option is organizing group outdoor activities, like hiking or cycling, which provide an opportunity to enjoy nature while staying active. These activities encourage social interaction and physical movement, both of which are beneficial for your gut.

Or, if you're more comfortable online, forums and support groups can be great places to connect with others who share similar health goals, and many places offer online classes. These connections can be invaluable, offering both emotional support and practical advice as you travel along your health journey.

On the flip side, loneliness can really take a toll on your gut health. Studies have shown that social isolation can disrupt the gut microbiome, leading to an increase in harmful bacteria and a decrease in beneficial ones. It's a reminder that we're social creatures by nature, and our bodies function best when we're connected to others. Isolation can lead to increased stress and anxiety, further exacerbating digestive issues. It's like trying to tend a garden without sunlight; without the warmth of social interaction, our health can wither. Making an effort to reach out and connect with others can counteract these effects, supporting not just your mental health but your gut as well.

As we wrap up this chapter, it's clear that lifestyle changes play an important role in supporting gut health. Next, we'll explore how to overcome common gut health challenges, equipping you with the tools to address any obstacles along the way.

4
OVERCOMING COMMON GUT HEALTH CHALLENGES

Have you ever felt your belly swell like a balloon after a meal, or found yourself stifling a burp in a quiet room? You're not alone. Bloating and gas are common challenges, and they often leave us feeling uncomfortable and self-conscious. As discussed earlier, these symptoms can be your body's way of signaling that something isn't quite right. Understanding the causes is the first step in addressing them. One of the major culprits is a group of carbohydrates known as FODMAPs, which stands for fermentable oligosaccharides, disaccharides, monosaccharides, and polyols. These are found in foods like onions, garlic, beans, and certain fruits and can be difficult for some people to digest, leading to fermentation in the gut and, consequently, gas and bloating. Fast eating and carbonated beverages can also contribute by introducing excess air into your digestive system.

When you eat quickly, you tend to swallow more air, which can accumulate in your stomach like an inflatable pool toy. We talked about mindful eating in the previous chapter and the importance of chewing slowly, and this is another reason why. Similarly, fizzy drinks release carbon dioxide in your stomach, adding to the gas. These habits may seem harmless, but they can exacerbate discomfort. So, how do we tackle these pesky symptoms? One effective strategy is to practice mindful eating, as mentioned earlier, and by also incorporating digestive aids like ginger or peppermint tea into your diet. Both are known for their soothing properties, helping to relax your digestive muscles and reduce gas production.

Your gut bacteria also play a significant role in gas production. As these microbes break down undigested food in the colon, they produce gas as a byproduct. This natural process is a sign that your gut is hard at work, so having gas is not an issue. However, an imbalance in your gut microbiome can lead to excessive gas, especially when certain bacteria overproduce it. Balancing your microbiome with a healthy diet and possibly probiotics can help regulate this process, reducing bloating and discomfort.

Sometimes, these strategies aren't enough, and that's when it might be time to seek professional advice. Persistent or severe symptoms that interfere with daily life should not be ignored. If you're experiencing significant weight loss or symptoms like anemia, it's highly advisable to consult a healthcare professional. These could be signs of a more serious underlying condition that requires medical attention. A doctor can help determine the root cause and recommend appropriate treatments or dietary adjustments.

Over to You! It's Time to Reflect...

Take a moment to observe your eating habits over the next few days. Are you eating quickly or reaching for fizzy drinks regularly? Keep a journal to track how these habits affect your digestion—experiment with eating more slowly and swapping carbonated beverages for herbal teas. Reflect on any changes in your symptoms and overall comfort.

LEAKY GUT: UNDERSTANDING AND HEALING

You have already learned a bit about the leaky gut. Imagine your gut lining as a fine sieve, selectively allowing nutrients to pass into your bloodstream while keeping out harmful substances. As you now know, when this lining becomes overly permeable—a condition often referred to as "leaky gut"—it can lead to chaos. Increased intestinal permeability means that toxins, microbes, and undigested food particles might slip through the cracks, entering the bloodstream and potentially triggering inflammation throughout the body. This inflammation is like an uninvited guest that overstays its welcome, contributing to a range of issues from digestive disorders to more systemic symptoms like fatigue and joint pain. While "leaky gut syndrome" isn't officially recognized as a medical diagnosis, its impact on health can be significant, especially for those already dealing with conditions like IBS or autoimmune diseases.

Several factors can contribute to the development of a leaky gut, and chronic stress is a major player. When stress becomes a constant companion, the body produces excess cortisol, a hormone that can weaken the gut lining over time. Stress can be a little like a relentless wave, eroding the sandcastle walls of your gut's defenses. A diet high in processed foods and sugars can also exacerbate this condition. These foods often lack the nutrients necessary to support gut health and can feed harmful bacteria, leading to dysbiosis. It's like fueling your car with the wrong type of gasoline—eventually, the engine will sputter and fail. Embracing a diet rich in whole, unprocessed foods, however, can provide the nutrients needed to support a healthy gut lining and fend off inflammation.

As you're figuring out, there's a lot you can do to improve your gut and support gut barrier repair. For example, incorporating bone broth and collagen-rich foods is one effective approach. These foods provide essential amino acids that can help rebuild gut lining integrity. Think of collagen as the scaffolding that supports your gut's architecture, patching up the gaps caused by increased permeability. Eliminating processed and inflammatory foods is equally important. By removing these culprits, you give your gut the chance to heal without constant irritation. Focus on nourishing your body with anti-inflammatory foods like leafy greens, berries, and healthy fats. This shift can help create an ideal environment where your gut can thrive.

In addition to dietary changes, certain supplements may aid in healing a leaky gut. L-glutamine, an amino acid, is often recommended for its role in repairing the intestinal lining. Probiotics, we know, can be highly beneficial, acting as peacekeepers and maintaining harmony within your gut's ecosystem.

The complexities of a leaky gut can feel overwhelming at first, but understanding its triggers and potential solutions offers a healthier path forward.

FOOD SENSITIVITIES AND ALLERGIES: DISCOVERING WHAT WORKS FOR YOU

Think back to a time when you ate something and felt unwell afterward. Maybe you experienced a bout of bloating, a stomach ache, or a sudden rash? It's possible you were dealing with a food sensitivity or allergy. These two conditions, though often confused, are quite different. A food allergy involves an immune system response; your body mistakenly identifies a harmless food protein as a threat and reacts defensively. This can lead to severe reactions like hives or even anaphylaxis, which demands immediate medical attention.

On the other hand, food sensitivities typically don't involve the immune system. They occur when your body struggles to digest certain foods, leading to discomfort like bloating, headaches, stomach pain, or skin rashes. While not life-threatening, sufferers know very well that sensitivities can significantly impact their quality of life.

Identifying whether you have a food sensitivity or allergy can be a bit of a detective mission, but one worth embarking on and finding once and for all, what the issue is. Symptoms of sensitivities, such as digestive troubles or skin irritations, can appear hours or even days after consuming the offending food, making it tricky to pinpoint the cause. Elimination diets can be helpful. By systematically removing suspected foods and then reintroducing them one at a time, you can observe how your body reacts. Keeping a food journal during this process is invaluable, as suggested earlier, as it helps track what you eat and how you feel, revealing patterns you might otherwise miss. For allergies, professional allergy tests conducted by a healthcare provider can offer clear answers. These tests can identify specific allergens, providing a roadmap for what to avoid.

Managing life with food sensitivities or allergies requires a strategic approach, especially when it comes to diet, but the effort will pay off. Start by mastering the art of reading food labels! Ingredients like gluten, dairy, or nuts can hide in unexpected places, so you'll need to become a label detective. Understanding cross-contamination risks is equally important; even trace amounts of allergens can trigger a reaction in some people.

Finding suitable alternatives is key, too. If dairy is an issue, explore plant-based milks like almond or oat milk. For those avoiding gluten, grains like rice or quinoa offer excellent substitutes. Don't hesitate to experiment with new recipes and products to keep your meals exciting and aligned with your dietary needs.

Working with healthcare professionals can make a world of difference here too. Nutritionists and allergists bring expertise to the table, helping you work through the complexities of food sensitivities and allergies. A dietitian can suggest balanced meal plans that ensure you're getting essential nutrients without triggering symptoms.

Over to You! It's Time to Reflect…

Textual Element: Case Study

Consider Jodie, who struggled with undiagnosed food sensitivities for years. By working closely with a nutritionist, she identified dairy and gluten as her main triggers. With her dietitian's help, she crafted a meal plan filled with delicious alternatives that kept her symptoms at bay, which basically changed her life! Emily's story highlights the importance of professional guidance in managing food sensitivities.

Take a moment to think about whether you may like to reach out to a professional for guidance, and if so, what would you ask them. Now is a good time to start a list of questions you may like to ask a professional.

THE ROLE OF ANTIBIOTICS AND GUT RECOVERY

Antibiotics are often hailed as medical marvels, essential for fighting off infections that could otherwise become life-threatening, and they can really get us back on track when feeling quite ill. However, as you may have heard, they unfortunately come with their own set of challenges, particularly for your gut health. The problem is that when antibiotics enter your system, they don't discriminate; they target bad bacteria but also wipe out beneficial ones. This reduction in beneficial bacteria can upset the delicate balance within your gut microbiome. The absence of these beneficial bacteria leaves room for opportunistic pathogens to move in, often leading to digestive issues and a compromised immune system.

Sometimes, antibiotics can't be avoided, so once you've completed a course of antibiotics, the road to gut recovery begins. The first step is reintroducing probiotics into your diet. These live microorganisms, such as yogurt, kefir, and fermented vegetables can help replenish the beneficial bacteria that antibiotics wipe out. You can also consider taking a high-quality probiotic supplement, but make sure to choose one with multiple strains and a high count of colony-forming units (CFUs) for maximum effectiveness. Alongside probiotics, incorporating prebiotic-rich foods is equally crucial because, as we covered earlier, prebiotics are essentially the food that nourishes your good bacteria, helping them thrive. Foods like bananas, asparagus, and oats are excellent choices to support microbial growth.

Using antibiotics judiciously is vital for maintaining long-term gut health. Avoiding unnecessary prescriptions can help protect your gut's natural balance, so it's essential to consult with a healthcare provider to determine whether antibiotics are truly necessary for your condition. Sometimes, a narrow-spectrum antibiotic, which targets specific bacteria, can be used instead of a broad-spectrum one, minimizing the collateral damage to your gut flora.

Repeated antibiotic use can have lasting implications for your gut health. Over time, frequent courses of antibiotics may increase your susceptibility to infections and digestive issues. This is because, with each course, your gut loses some of its resilience, becoming less capable of bouncing back to its original, healthy state. Studies have shown that certain beneficial bacteria may never fully return, leaving a permanent gap in your microbial defenses. This can lead to a cycle where your gut becomes more prone to imbalances, requiring further interventions.

So, understanding the impact of antibiotics on your gut is essential for making informed health decisions when considering taking antibiotics.

GUT HEALTH IN THE MODERN WORLD: BALANCING WELLNESS WITH LIFE'S DEMANDS

With our increasingly busy lives these days, maintaining gut health amidst the demands of a modern lifestyle can seem like just another thing to add to the juggle. Our lives are often fast-paced, filled with responsibilities that leave little room for self-care. We also find ourselves seated for long hours, whether at a desk job or in front of a screen, with little time to stretch our legs. This sedentary lifestyle can slow down our metabolism, impacting digestion and, in turn, our gut health. It's not just the inactivity; the rush of our daily routines often leads to hastily consumed meals, barely chewed before we move on to the next task. High-stress work environments further complicate things, and we know how stress can affect our digestive systems.

Yet, even with a packed schedule, there are ways to incorporate gut-friendly habits into your routine. Meal prepping, as mentioned earlier, can be a total lifesaver, ensuring that you have healthy, gut-friendly options on hand throughout the week.

Another simple yet effective habit is incorporating regular movement breaks during your workday. Set a timer to remind yourself to stand up, stretch, or walk around every hour. Not only does this keep your body active, but it also aids digestion by promoting regular bowel movements and reducing the sluggishness that can occur from sitting too long. You'll be doing your body a favor while also feeling refreshed when you get back to the desk.

It's also worth thinking about how our constant connectivity affects our gut health. We all know that the screens we rely on can be both a blessing and a curse. However, excessive screen time, especially before meals or bedtime, can disrupt our body's natural rhythms. Try reducing screen exposure at these critical times. Instead of scrolling through your phone during lunch, take the opportunity to eat mindfully, focusing on your food and its flavors. Digital detoxes, even short ones, can be refreshing. Consider using mindfulness apps to help you disconnect and center yourself, even if just for a few minutes a day. This practice can reduce stress and improve your mental well-being, indirectly benefiting your gut.

Take, for example, the story of Laura, a marketing executive who successfully integrated gut health practices into her hectic lifestyle. Despite her demanding job, she found time for evening yoga sessions that helped her unwind and keep stress at bay. These sessions not only improved her flexibility but also supported her digestive health. Laura also started meal prepping on Sundays, making a week's worth of nutrient-rich meals that kept her energized and focused. Her commitment to these small changes reaped significant rewards, demonstrating that with a bit of planning, even the busiest among us can make room for better health.

Balancing gut health with modern demands doesn't require a complete lifestyle overhaul. Small, sustainable changes can fit into your life and can support your gut health even amidst the chaos.

TRUSTING THE PROCESS: OVERCOMING DOUBTS ON YOUR GUT HEALTH JOURNEY

It's not uncommon to approach gut health with a fair dose of skepticism. After all, the market is flooded with products and advice that promise miraculous results. Probiotics, for example, often claim to be the cure-all for digestive woes. While they offer significant benefits, the truth is more nuanced. The efficacy of probiotics can vary based on the strains used and the individual taking them. Some people experience dramatic improvements, while others notice little change. It's therefore essential to understand that while probiotics can be beneficial, they're not a one-size-fits-all solution. Their effectiveness depends on your unique gut environment and health needs. This is why it's vital to approach gut health practices with an open mind, backed by evidence-based information.

I'm sure at this point in this book, you're understanding that a tailored approach to gut health is critical. Just as we all have different fingerprints, our gut microbiomes are unique. Personalizing your dietary choices and lifestyle habits can make a significant difference in your health outcomes. Instead of following generic advice, think about working with a healthcare professional who can guide you in understanding your body's specific needs. They can help tailor strategies that align with your personal health conditions, whether it's adjusting your diet to manage IBS symptoms or incorporating stress-reducing activities to balance your hormones. Personalization is about listening to your body and responding to its cues, giving you the knowledge and confidence to make informed decisions that lead to lasting change.

Building confidence in your gut health decisions involves trusting your instincts and taking a proactive role in your well-being. You've already begun to educate yourself about how the gut works and how different foods and habits can affect it. This self-education can also come from reading reputable sources, attending workshops, or even participating in online courses. The more you understand, the better equipped you'll be to make choices that align with your health goals. Remember, you're the expert on your body. Trust your gut—literally and figuratively—and don't be afraid to challenge conventional wisdom if it doesn't resonate with you.

For those keen on further exploration, a wealth of resources awaits. Check out reading lists that cover the latest research and developments in gut health. Books, articles, and scientific journals offer a more thorough understanding of the complexities of our digestive systems. Online support groups can also be invaluable. Connecting with others who share similar experiences can provide a boost of encouragement and practical tips. Additionally, keeping in contact with health professionals ensures you have ongoing guidance and support. Whether it's a nutritionist, a GI specialist, or a holistic health coach, these professionals can offer insights and adjustments that keep you on track.

As we wrap up this chapter, remember that the path to wellness is unique for each of us. By trusting your instincts, educating yourself, and seeking support when needed, you can achieve a balanced and healthy gut.

Note: At the end of the book, you'll find a resource guide for further discovery!

BE A GUT HEALTH ADVOCATE AND FRIEND:
YOUR REVIEW MAKES A POSITIVE DIFFERENCE

"Helping one person might not change the whole world, but it could change the world for one person."

— UNKNOWN

Would you help someone just like you? Someone looking to improve their gut health or someone curious about the gut-body connection, but is unsure where to start?

But to reach more people, I need your help.

Most people choose books based on reviews. So, I'm asking you to help a fellow wellness explorer by leaving a review.

It costs nothing and takes less than a minute, yet it could transform someone's journey to achieving a happier, healthier gut. Your review could help...

...one more person understand how to nurture their family's digestion and well-being.
...one more friend discover how to balance their gut for vibrant health inside and out.
...one more family learn how personalized gut health can keep them thriving together.
...one more small business empower their community with gut-friendly food options.
...one more dream of achieving lasting gut health come true.

To make a difference, simply scan the QR code below and leave a review:

[https://www.amazon.com/review/review-your-purchases/?asin=BOOKASIN]

If you enjoy helping others, you're definitely my kind of person. Thank you so much, and take care!

Ellody Kamp

5
CREATING YOUR UNIQUE GUT HEALTH PLAN

If you're been completing the journal reflections up to this point (if not, you may like to head back and try them out), then you'll be aware of what foods trigger specific reactions, how stress affects you physically, and how trying out various things like eating more fiber, including probiotics etc., into your diet and lifestyle have improved your gut health.

Self-Assessment Tools: Understanding Your Gut Needs

If you're still having trouble figuring out what is the cause of certain symptoms, online quizzes and surveys can be great tools to gauge your current gut health. These quizzes often ask questions about your diet, lifestyle habits, and any symptoms you might be experiencing. They provide a general overview, highlighting areas that may need attention.

Technology has become an invaluable ally in the quest for personalized health insights. Apps designed to track food intake and symptoms offer a convenient way to monitor how different factors affect your gut. You can easily and quickly log meals, note any reactions, and even track your mood and stress levels. This data can reveal trends that might otherwise go unnoticed. Wearable devices add another layer of insight, measuring physical activity and stress, which we know impact digestion.

Despite the benefits of self-assessment, there are times when professional guidance is needed. If you experience persistent or unexplained digestive symptoms, it's important to consult a healthcare professional. They can provide a comprehensive analysis and recommend appropriate testing, such as microbiome assessments that analyze the types and quantities of microorganisms in your gut. Though these tests aren't diagnostic, they offer a deeper understanding of your gut's ecosystem.

SETTING REALISTIC GOALS FOR GUT HEALTH TRANSFORMATION

Setting clear goals can be a game-changer when you're working on improving your gut health because, without a clear endpoint, it's easy to feel lost or overwhelmed, or even be tempted to give up. By defining what success looks like for you, whether it's reducing bloating or increasing energy levels, you give yourself a target to aim for. This clarity helps transform vague intentions into actionable steps.

It's important to remind yourself here that you need to strike a balance between ambition and realism. While it's great to dream big (I love that!), setting too many goals at once can be daunting. Instead, you can try dividing your goals into short-term and long-term categories. Short-term goals might be all about introducing more high-fiber foods into your diet, while long-term goals could include achieving a consistent exercise routine that supports gut health. There's no rush, and it's always better to take it one step at a time rather than go too hard and then feel overwhelmed in the process and give up!

Creating productive goals requires a thoughtful approach. I've found that the SMART framework is a reliable method that ensures goals are well-defined and achievable. SMART stands for Specific, Measurable, Achievable, Relevant, and Time-bound. For example, instead of saying, "I want to eat healthier," you could set a SMART goal like "Increase my fiber intake by 5 grams per day over the next month." This approach not only provides a clear target but also allows you to track your progress and make adjustments along the way. By focusing on each component of the SMART criteria, I'm confident that you will set yourself up for success! Basically, this process transforms what might seem like an overwhelming task into a more manageable and rewarding one.

Life is dynamic, and so are your goals! As you make progress, take a few moments to reevaluate and adjust your goals to reflect your current situation. Perhaps you've reached your initial goal of increasing fiber intake, and now you're ready to focus on improving your physical activity or reducing stress. It's essential to recognize that our needs change over time, and our goals should adapt accordingly. Reassessing your goals every few months can help you stay aligned with your evolving priorities. Don't beat yourself up if you slip up or get behind in your goals. Life events, like a new job or moving to a new city, can impact your routine and require adjustments and a flexible mindset. Being open to these changes makes sure that your goals remain relevant and achievable, supporting your ongoing gut-health journey.

We've already chatted about celebrating milestones along the way, but it won't hurt to remind you here again. No matter how small the achievement is, each positive step can provide a motivational boost and reinforce positive behaviors. Why not set up a reward system for reaching significant goals? It doesn't have to be extravagant—maybe treating yourself to a new book, enjoying a leisurely day at the park, or a purchase you've had your eye on. Sharing your successes with a supportive network, too, whether it's friends, family, or an online community, can amplify the joy of your accomplishments. You'll inspire others too, which is a wonderful thing. These celebrations boost morale and create a positive feedback loop, encouraging continued progress and commitment to your health goals.

In the end, setting realistic goals for gut health transformation means creating a path that aligns with your needs and aspirations. It's exciting, isn't it?!

GUT HEALTH AT EVERY AGE: ADAPTING PRACTICES FOR EVERY LIFE STAGE

As we move through different phases of life, our bodies undergo changes that can significantly impact our gut health. Recognizing these shifts is just so crucial for maintaining a balanced digestive system.

Each life stage brings its own set of challenges and needs when it comes to gut health.

Adolescents, for instance, experience rapid growth spurts that demand higher nutritional intake. This period often sees a shift in dietary habits as teens explore their independence, sometimes opting for convenience over nutrition. Encouraging a balanced diet rich in fiber, protein, and healthy fats can support their developing bodies and gut health.

For adults, juggling career and family responsibilities can lead to irregular eating habits and increased stress, both of which can affect digestion. It's therefore important to prioritize regular meals, stress management, and perhaps a probiotic supplement to keep the gut in check.

For older adults, there's an increased need for dietary fiber and hydration. As we age, the digestive system slows down, and the gut may not absorb nutrients as efficiently. So, fiber-rich foods like whole grains, fruits, and vegetables become even more necessary in promoting regular bowel movements and preventing constipation. Staying hydrated is equally vital, as it helps fiber do its job and keeps the digestive tract functioning smoothly. Making these dietary adjustments can help older adults maintain gut health and an overall sense of feeling great and full of energy.

Each stage requires a tailored approach that considers the unique demands on the body and lifestyle.

Life transitions can also play a significant role in gut health. Take pregnancy, for example, when hormonal changes can slow digestion and increase the need for certain nutrients. Pregnant individuals often find that their gut health needs shift, such as requiring more fiber to combat constipation and an increased focus on hydration. Postpartum, the body undergoes further changes as it recovers and adjusts to new routines. During these times, it's helpful to focus on nutrient-dense foods and possibly consult with a healthcare provider for personalized advice.

PERIMENOPAUSE AND THE GUT-HORMONE CONNECTION

As women approach the transitional phase of perimenopause, the body undergoes significant changes, not just in the obvious areas like hormones and reproductive health, but also within the intricate ecosystem of the gut. This intersection of gut health and hormonal fluctuation unveils a fascinating and lesser-known relationship, drawing focus on the estrobolome—the key player in this symbiotic dance.

The estrobolome is a subset of the gut microbiota tasked with regulating oestrogen metabolism. As oestrogen levels fluctuate during perimenopause, the estrobolome adjusts, potentially altering the balance of microbes and influencing overall gut health.

Emerging research paints a picture of reduced microbial diversity during this phase—a shift that could lead to a microbiome more similar to that of men, deviating from the diverse landscape typically seen in pre-menopausal women. This transformation has implications not only for digestive health but also for systemic well-being, as gut microbes can significantly impact mood and metabolic functions. And this makes sense because women are finding their moods fluctuating a lot during this time in their lives, as well as reporting being unable to tolerate foods they were previously able to, such as chili. Many woman also find they cannot tolerate alcohol as they used to, as their body struggles to process it.

Hormones like estradiol do double-duty, limiting intestinal permeability and safeguarding the gut barrier. With their decline, the fortress of the gut might face vulnerabilities, and new issues like food intolerances (as mentioned above) and IBS may appear, although scientific consensus is still forming.

So, how can women harness these insights to bolster their gut health during perimenopause? The answer lies in dietary diversity. Really taking the time to incorporate a rainbow of fruits, vegetables, whole grains, and nuts can fuel the gut's beneficial bacteria. Probiotics emerge as another ally, offering a gentle nudge towards microbial harmony.

Ultimately, as general practitioners increasingly recognize the gut's role in overall health, they can guide women through perimenopause with tailored dietary strategies. If their local GP is not experienced with menopause symptoms (and many are not as yet), then consider speaking to a specialist or nutritionist who can help point you in the right direction. This is not a time for 'sucking it up' and accepting this discomfort (which can sometimes be highly debilitating, especially of the mood fluctuations are extreme) but a time to advocate for their support. By doing so, women may not only ease the symptoms of this life stage but also set a foundation for healthier years beyond.

Similarly, retirement marks another transition, often accompanied by shifts in daily routines. This period can be an opportunity to reassess diet and incorporate more movement, both of which can benefit gut health.

This brings us to the story of Carmel, a retiree who found her digestion lagging as she settled into a less active lifestyle. She began incorporating daily walks and increased her intake of fruits and vegetables, which improved her gut health and boosted her energy. These simple changes made a big difference.

Then there's Max, a teenager who struggled with gut issues during his growth spurts. With guidance, he learned to balance his diet with more whole foods (and resisting the processed foods his friends were eating), which helped stabilize his digestion and supported his development.

These examples show that with awareness and adaptation, gut health can be managed successfully across various life stages.

INTEGRATING GUT HEALTH WITH OTHER WELLNESS GOALS

Think about how everything in your life is connected, much like pieces of a puzzle coming together to form a complete picture. We now know that when it comes to gut health, it's more than just digestion. We know that the gut-brain axis, a communication highway of nerves, hormones, and chemicals, links your gut with your mental state. We all therefore want a healthy gut that can lead to a clearer mind, reduced anxiety, and improved mood. It's like having a supportive friend within you, constantly working to keep your mind sharp and your spirit high!

So, we understand that eating the right foods and taking care of our mental health will affect our gut, and vice versa. Now we want you to think about how you can move your body more in order to support your gut health too. Integrating gut-friendly foods into your fitness nutrition plan will fuel your workouts and optimize your body's performance during your workout and subsequent recovery. Foods rich in fiber and probiotics can enhance your gut microbiome, which in turn supports muscle recovery and energy levels. As you build your fitness routine, consider incorporating meals that are not only high in protein but also packed with nutrients that promote gut health. This approach will help ensure that your body is not only strong but also balanced and capable of handling the physical demands you place on it. Because there's no point in keeping fit and doing tough workouts if your body doesn't have the fuel to sustain or recover from them. We need to think about creating a harmony where nutrition and fitness work hand in hand, supporting each other for better results.

A balanced wellness routine will help you achieve holistic health. Start by scheduling regular exercise sessions, whether it's a brisk walk, a yoga class, or a gym workout. Physical activity is known to stimulate the production of short-chain fatty acids in the gut, which have anti-inflammatory properties and support gut health. Ideally, pair this with relaxation techniques like meditation or deep breathing exercises, which can reduce stress and its negative impact on your gut.

Ensuring adequate sleep is another pillar of this routine. Quality sleep is essential for your body to repair and rejuvenate, including your gut. It's during sleep that your body does a lot of its healing work, keeping your gut running smoothly.

To see this in action, consider a weekly wellness plan (tweaked to suit your preferences and lifestyle) such as the following:

- Start your week with a meal prep session, focusing on gut-friendly foods like fermented vegetables, whole grains, and lean proteins.
- Schedule workouts you enjoy, whether that's a morning walk or an evening Pilates class.
- Incorporate mindfulness practices, perhaps a morning meditation or an evening gratitude journal, to foster a sense of peace and focus.
- Engage in community activities that can also provide social support, which is beneficial for both mental health and gut wellness. Joining a local cooking class or a fitness group can offer camaraderie and motivation, making your wellness routine more enjoyable and sustainable. Monitor your progress across these goals to understand how these elements work together to improve your well-being.

- Regular check-ins with a wellness coach or support group can provide guidance and encouragement, helping you stay on track and make adjustments as needed. These interactions offer a wealth of knowledge and camaraderie, reinforcing your commitment to a healthier, more balanced life.

Over to You! It's Time to Reflect...

How have changes in your life stage impacted your gut health? What specific nutritional or lifestyle adjustments do you think would benefit you now? If you're in a transition phase, like pregnancy or menopause, how can you actively support your evolving gut health needs through diet and lifestyle changes?

Next, we'll explore the exciting world of expanding your gut health knowledge, looking at some global practices and innovations that can further improve your wellness path.

6

EXPANDING YOUR GUT HEALTH KNOWLEDGE

Every culture has its own relationship with food, and these traditions often hold valuable insights into gut health. For example, think of a beautiful Mediterranean table, where meals are a celebration of life, filled with vibrant colors and robust flavors. This diet is rich in whole grains, fresh vegetables, and healthy fats like olive oil and nuts. This is more than eating delicious food; it's a lifestyle that cherishes the quality and enjoyment of food. The Mediterranean diet, well-known for its benefits, focuses on foods that naturally support a healthy gut, including fiber-rich vegetables and omega-3 fatty acids from fish. This approach to eating is about balance and pleasure, making it easy to see why it's linked to lower rates of heart disease and improved gut health.

Travel eastward, and you'll find the influence of fermentation in Asian diets. Think about the complex, spicy tang of kimchi or the subtle earthiness of natto. These fermented foods are staples in countries like Korea and Japan, and they offer a natural source of probiotics. We know that including fermented foods in your diet can be a simple yet effective way to improve gut health, but the beauty of these foods is that they enhance both flavor and health.

Beyond food, ancient medicinal systems like Ayurveda and Traditional Chinese Medicine offer some fantastic insights into gut health. Ayurveda, a holistic system from India, focuses on digestive balance through doshas—energetic forces that govern physiological activity. This approach is all about the importance of digestive fire, or "Agni," which is believed to be essential for health. In Ayurveda, maintaining a strong Agni is fundamental for nutrient absorption and overall vitality. Similarly, Traditional Chinese Medicine uses herbs and dietary adjustments to support digestive health, viewing digestion as central to energy balance and well-being. These systems encourage a deep connection with our bodies, promoting harmony between diet, lifestyle, and internal balance.

Cultural attitudes towards eating also provide valuable lessons. Take the French, for example, who are known for their mindful approach to meals. Eating in France is a leisurely affair, focusing on quality over quantity. This mindful eating practice supports digestion and enhances meal enjoyment. The French really know how to savor each bite, appreciate the flavors, and connect with those around them. Indigenous cultures also offer wisdom, often focused on natural remedies and plant-based diets. These perspectives highlight the importance of traditional knowledge and natural ingredients in maintaining health. By observing these cultural practices, we can learn so much and begin to view food not just as fuel or for our taste buds, but as a basis of good health and community connection.

Why not have some fun experimenting with global recipes that use fermented foods or whole grains and observe how your body responds? Consider adopting meal timing strategies from different cultures, such as eating your largest meal at midday, which aligns with Ayurvedic principles. These practices can complement your existing routines, offering new ways to nourish your body and support your gut. Embracing global wisdom can enrich your understanding of health, providing diverse tools to foster a balanced, vibrant life.

Over to You! It's Time to Reflect...

Global Recipe Exploration

Challenge yourself to try a new recipe from a different culture each week. Start with a Mediterranean dish rich in whole grains and healthy fats, then move on to a Korean recipe featuring kimchi. Keep a journal to note how these foods affect your digestion and overall well-being. Reflect on the experience of cooking and eating these global dishes, and consider incorporating your favorites into your regular meal rotation.

THE FUTURE OF GUT HEALTH: BREAKTHROUGHS AND INNOVATIONS ON THE HORIZON

It's exciting to see the world of gut health rapidly evolving, with research revealing new ways to boost our well-being. One remarkable development is microbiome transplant therapy, an innovative approach to restoring balance in the gut. By transplanting healthy microbiota from one individual to another, these therapies offer hope for those struggling with chronic gut issues. Fascinating, isn't it?! This process, often called fecal microbiota transplantation (FMT), has shown promise in treating conditions like Clostridioides difficile infections, which can be resistant to standard treatments. Imagine the potential of restoring balance in your gut by introducing a community of beneficial bacteria that can outcompete harmful strains. It's like resetting your gut flora to a healthier state, allowing your body to function more efficiently.

We touched on the idea earlier of personalized nutrition, which is also gaining traction, thanks to advances in gut microbiome profiling. By analyzing your unique microbiome, researchers can tailor dietary recommendations to support your specific health needs. This approach considers the complex interplay between diet and gut flora, offering a more targeted way to address particular health issues. It would indeed be amazing and life-changing to know exactly which foods will best support your gut health and change your diet accordingly.

Advancements in technology are also pushing along gut health research and practice. Home testing kits for microbiome analysis are becoming more accessible, allowing you to gain insights into your gut health from the comfort of your home. Amazing! These kits can provide valuable information about the diversity and composition of your gut microbiota, helping you make informed decisions about your diet and lifestyle. Additionally, artificial intelligence is being used to predict gut health outcomes, offering a glimpse into the future of personalized medicine. By analyzing vast amounts of data, AI can identify patterns and correlations that might not be immediately apparent, providing a deeper understanding of how various factors influence gut health.

Targeted probiotics are being developed to address specific imbalances, offering a more precise way to support gut health. These probiotics are designed to enhance the growth of beneficial bacteria while suppressing harmful strains, creating a more balanced gut environment. Prebiotic fibers are also being engineered to stimulate the development of specific bacteria, further refining our approach to gut health. By understanding the unique needs of your microbiome, these advancements offer a more nuanced way to promote digestive wellness.

As you can see, the implications of these innovations for future health strategies are immense! Integrating gut health into preventive healthcare models could revolutionize how we approach wellness, shifting the focus from treating symptoms to optimizing health and focusing on prevention rather than cure. By addressing gut imbalances early, we may reduce the incidence of chronic diseases and improve overall vitality and health. Moreover, personalized interventions have the potential to reduce healthcare costs by offering targeted solutions that prevent the progression of health issues. This approach emphasizes the importance of understanding the complex relationships between diet, lifestyle, and gut health, offering a holistic path to wellness that is both effective and sustainable.

I understand that welcoming these advancements requires an open mind and a willingness to explore new possibilities. But as technology and research continue to evolve, the potential for improving our gut health and overall wellness expands. By staying informed and proactive, you can feel positive that the future of gut health is bright, offering many opportunities to optimize your health in ways we never thought possible.

GUT HEALTH MYTHS AND MISCONCEPTIONS

There's a lot of buzz around gut health these days, and with it comes a fair share of myths and misconceptions. One of the most common myths that we addressed earlier is that probiotics are a cure-all for digestive issues and that not all probiotic strains are created equal, and their effects can vary significantly from person to person. It's essential to understand that probiotics work best as part of a balanced diet and lifestyle, rather than a standalone solution. Relying solely on them without addressing other aspects of health, like diet and stress, might leave you feeling underwhelmed by the results.

Another widespread misconception is that a gluten-free diet is beneficial for everyone. It's easy to see why this myth persists, given the popularity of gluten-free products and diets. However, unless you have celiac disease or a diagnosed gluten intolerance, cutting out gluten might not provide any health benefits at all. In fact, gluten-containing whole grains can be an excellent source of fiber, which supports gut health. Eliminating these grains without a valid reason can lead to nutrient deficiencies. It's important, therefore, to remember that dietary choices should reflect individual needs, rather than following trends without understanding their impact.

Then there are the misunderstandings around food intolerances and allergies, where food allergies involve an immune response and can be life-threatening. At the same time, intolerances tend to cause digestive discomfort but aren't dangerous. Similarly, many people view fat in the diet negatively, despite its essential role in health. Healthy fats, like those found in avocados and nuts, are not only vital for hormone production and nutrient absorption but also support feelings of fullness. They aren't the enemy; rather, they're a key component of a balanced diet.

Misinformation often stems from marketing and social media. Unfortunately, many products are marketed with exaggerated claims, promising miraculous results that lack scientific backing. Social media platforms can amplify these messages, spreading them quickly and widely. Additionally, non-experts sometimes misinterpret scientific studies, leading to further confusion. For instance, a study on a specific population might not apply to everyone, yet it can be presented as a universal truth. Being aware of these sources of misinformation helps in making more informed choices about your health.

To sail through this sea of information safely, it's necessary to critically assess the credibility of the sources you encounter. Look for information from reputable organizations and peer-reviewed studies. If unsure, check the expertise of the person providing advice—are they a qualified healthcare professional or a self-proclaimed expert? Remember, it's okay to question and seek clarification. Reaching out to professionals, such as registered dietitians or doctors, can provide personalized guidance based on your unique health needs, and you can have peace of mind that the advice is based on solid experience and credentials. They can help you sift through the noise, offering evidence-based recommendations that align with your goals. In a world filled with information, be a discerning consumer and take charge of your gut health with confidence.

THE ROLE OF GENETICS IN GUT HEALTH

When you think about gut health, genes might not be the first thing that comes to mind. But they actually play a key role in shaping your gut microbiome. Genetics can influence everything from how you digest food to your susceptibility to certain gut disorders! For example, if you've ever wondered why some people seem to handle spicy foods like jalapeños without a problem while others can't, genes could be a part of the answer. Your genetic makeup can affect how your body processes nutrients and how well it can fend off inflammation. Genetic predispositions can also make you more prone to conditions like irritable bowel syndrome (IBS), where specific gene variants have been linked to increased risk. These genetic factors are like the invisible strings that pull the levers on how your gut functions, highlighting the intricate relationship between your genes and digestion.

Recent genomic studies have shed some interesting light on just how much genetics influences the gut. Through research, scientists have identified specific gene variants associated with IBS, which opens the door to better understanding and potentially managing this common condition. If you knew that your IBS symptoms have a genetic component, it could explain why certain treatments work better for you than others.

Studies have also revealed the heritability of certain microbiome traits, meaning that the composition of your gut flora can be influenced by your genes. This means that if your parents have a diverse and balanced microbiome, you might inherit similar traits, giving you a head start in maintaining good gut health. These findings show us the importance of considering genetic factors when learning about gut health, as they provide a more comprehensive understanding of what makes your gut unique.

The potential for genetic interventions in gut health is an exciting frontier. With advancements in genetic research, the possibility of gene-based therapies for digestive conditions is becoming more tangible. Imagine a future where you could receive treatments specifically designed to address your genetic predispositions, offering a more targeted approach to managing gut health. Personalized dietary recommendations based on genetic profiles are also on the horizon. This customized approach moves beyond the generic dietary guidelines, offering a more nuanced and effective way to support your digestive system.

Take Ben, for example, who had a family history of heart disease and made changes to his diet and lifestyle to prioritize his gut health. By eating more whole foods and doing some regular exercise, he noticed improvements in his cholesterol levels and overall cardiovascular health. We, too, with a bit of knowledge, can change our diet to prevent or manage chronic diseases.

7
DELICIOUS & PRACTICAL: RECIPES TO BOOST YOUR GUT HEALTH

Okay, let's jump further into some delicious and gut-friendly meal ideas, starting with waking up in the morning when your body feels energized and your mind is clear and ready to tackle the day. This isn't just the stuff of dreams; it's the power of starting your day with a nutritious breakfast. Breakfast is often hailed as the most important meal of the day, and for good reason. It's like the jump-start your gut needs to set a positive tone for the hours ahead. A fiber-rich breakfast can do wonders for your digestion, helping to stabilize blood sugar levels and keep you feeling full and focused. A breakfast rich in fiber will also support long-term gut health.

Fiber acts as a natural regulator, managing blood sugar and cholesterol while encouraging regular bowel movements. Whole grains like oats and quinoa are your gut's best friends, offering a hearty dose of fiber with each serving. Oats, in particular, are versatile and easy to prepare, making them a staple in gut-friendly breakfasts. Pair them with probiotic-rich yogurt or kefir, and you've got a meal that not only satisfies but also supports the delicate balance of bacteria in your gut. So easy! These ingredients are easy to incorporate into your morning routine, providing a delicious way to boost your gut health from the get-go. Remember, when you nourish your gut first thing in the morning, you lay the groundwork for a day where your body and mind perform at their best.

Now, for some yummy breakfast recipes that you can whip up easily at home. Overnight oats with chia seeds and berries are a perfect example of a meal that requires minimal effort but offers maximum benefit. Simply combine oats, chia seeds, and your choice of milk in a jar, then top with fresh berries. Let it sit overnight, and by morning, you'll have a creamy, fiber-rich breakfast waiting for you. The chia seeds add an extra nutritional boost, providing omega-3 fatty acids and fiber. Another great option is quinoa porridge with almond milk and cinnamon. This dish is warm, comforting, and packed with protein and fiber, making it an ideal way to start your day. The cinnamon adds a pinch of natural sweetness while helping to regulate blood sugar levels.

For those mornings when time seems to slip away, having quick and nutritious options on hand can be a lifesaver. Prepping smoothie ingredients the night before can save precious minutes during a hectic morning or stop you from reaching for something less than ideal, or even worse, skipping breakfast! Simply blend your favorite fruits with a scoop of yogurt or kefir, and you'll have a gut-friendly breakfast ready in seconds. Smoothies are not only convenient but also customizable, allowing you to tailor them to your taste and nutritional needs. Alternatively, consider batch-cooking breakfast muffins with flaxseed over the weekend. These muffins are both portable and packed with fiber and healthy fats, making them perfect for busy mornings when you need to grab something on the go.

Over to You! It's Time to Reflect...

Recipe Reflection

Think about your current breakfast routine. Does it include any gut-friendly foods? Challenge yourself to try one new recipe from this chapter or another source each week. Keep a journal to note how these changes affect your energy levels, digestion, and overall mood. Reflect on which recipes work best for you and consider incorporating them into your regular rotation.

LUNCHTIME SOLUTIONS FOR DIGESTIVE WELLNESS

I think you know by now that lunch is an integral part of maintaining your gut health. We're all busy, so take the time for a well-balanced lunch that can sustain your energy levels and support digestion. It's time to banish that afternoon slump into a thing of the past! Aim for the right mix of nutrients to keep your body functioning smoothly. For example, include a balance of carbohydrates, proteins, and healthy fats to give your gut what it needs to thrive and keep you feeling energized until dinner time. The right combination can also stabilize blood sugar, prevent cravings, and keep you feeling satisfied longer.

When putting together a gut-friendly lunch, focus on ingredients that promote digestive health, like leafy greens and cruciferous vegetables. Kale, spinach, and broccoli are excellent choices for they are rich in fiber, vitamins, and minerals. Pair these with lean proteins like chicken or tofu, which provide the building blocks your body needs to repair and grow. Healthy fats from avocados or olive oil can add flavor and satiety, helping to absorb fat-soluble vitamins and regulate inflammation.

How about a refreshing lentil salad with spinach and avocado? The lentils offer a hearty dose of plant-based protein and fiber, while the creamy avocado provides those healthy fats. The spinach adds a fresh crunch, along with essential nutrients like iron and calcium. Another power-packed lunch could be grilled chicken with roasted sweet potatoes and broccoli. The chicken is a lean protein that supports muscle maintenance, while the sweet potatoes are a complex carbohydrate that provides sustained energy. Broccoli adds fiber and antioxidants to boost your body's defenses.

Packing a gut-healthy lunch for work or school doesn't have to be a hassle. Mason jars can be your best friend here, allowing you to layer salads in a way that keeps them fresh and crisp. Start with a base of leafy greens, add protein like chickpeas or grilled chicken, top with colorful vegetables, and finish with a dressing. When you're ready to eat, simply shake the jar to distribute the dressing evenly. Another tip is to include fermented sides like pickles or kimchi.

Over to You! It's Time to Reflect...

Consider your current lunch habits. Are you including a balance of fiber, protein, and healthy fats? Use this checklist to evaluate your lunch:

- *Leafy greens or cruciferous vegetables: Yes / No*
- *Lean protein: Yes / No*
- *Healthy fats: Yes / No*
- *Fermented side: Yes / No*

Aim to incorporate more of these elements into your meals. Reflect on how these changes affect your digestion and energy levels throughout the day.

DINNERS FOR A HAPPY GUT

As the day winds down, dinner becomes a chance to reset and prepare your body for a restful night. A gut-friendly dinner should, of course, be tasty but also plays a key role in evening metabolism and aids digestion, setting you up for restorative sleep. When your evening meal is balanced, it helps regulate your digestive system so that your body efficiently processes nutrients. The right dinner can also prevent late-night cravings and improve sleep quality by stabilizing blood sugar levels. It can be helpful to think of it as the final act of nourishment for the day, making your gut calm and your body ready to relax.

The ingredients you choose for dinner can make a world of difference, so aim to include fiber-rich legumes and whole grains to keep your digestive system running smoothly. These foods offer a steady release of energy and keep you feeling satisfied longer, reducing the temptation to snack late at night. Consider incorporating lentils or chickpeas into your meals; they're not only nutritious but also versatile, fitting into a variety of dishes. Pair these with anti-inflammatory herbs and spices like turmeric, ginger, and garlic. These ingredients help reduce inflammation and support gut health, making them perfect for a soothing evening meal.

One delicious option for dinner is baked salmon with turmeric-spiced quinoa. This dish combines the healthy fats of salmon with the fiber and protein of quinoa, creating a meal that's both satisfying and beneficial for your gut. The turmeric adds a warm, earthy flavor while providing anti-inflammatory benefits.

For a quick and easy option, a vegetable stir-fry with ginger and garlic can be both satisfying and nutritious. Use a variety of colorful vegetables to maximize the vitamin and mineral content.

The ginger and garlic not only enhance the taste but also aid digestion, creating a meal that's as healthy as it is delicious. These recipes offer a balance of protein, carbs, and fats, ensuring your body has everything it needs to function optimally.

As you can see, creating a satisfying and nutritious dinner doesn't have to be complicated. Focus on balancing your meal with the right mix of protein, carbohydrates, and healthy fats. Incorporate a variety of colorful vegetables into your meals; they provide essential nutrients and antioxidants that support overall health. It can help to think of your plate as a canvas, where each color represents a different vitamin or mineral. By eating a rainbow of foods, you ensure that your body receives a wide range of nutrients.

Over to You! It's Time to Reflect...

Consider your current dinner habits. Are you including anti-inflammatory herbs and spices, fiber-rich foods, whole grains? Use this checklist to evaluate your dinner:

- *Balanced meal of lean protein, carbohydrates, and healthy fats: Yes / No*
- *Lentils and/or beans: Yes / No*
- *Anti-inflammatory herbs and spices: Yes / No*
- *Colorful mix of vegetables: Yes / No*

SNACK SMARTER: GUT-HEALTHY OPTIONS

Snacks are notorious for being unhealthy because they're just so tempting to reach for something quick and easy, especially when we're busy. But how good would it be to reach for a snack and know it's not just filling a gap in your hunger but genuinely nourishing your gut? It's totally possible! Snacking, often dismissed as a mere bridge between meals, holds the potential to be a super source of nourishment with the right choices and just a little thought and planning.

Mindful snacking is about picking foods that are satisfying but also beneficial for your digestion. By changing your focus to gut-friendly snacks, you can maintain stable energy levels throughout the day and prevent those dreaded mid-afternoon slumps. These snacks can aid digestion, thanks to their fiber content and nutrient density, turning a simple munch into a mini health boost.

Consider the simplicity and satisfaction (and deliciousness!) of sliced apples paired with almond butter. Apples are high in fiber, particularly pectin, which acts as a prebiotic, feeding the good bacteria in your gut. Almond butter, rich in healthy fats and protein, adds a creamy contrast, making this snack not only delicious but also a powerhouse for your digestive health. For a savory option, try hummus with carrot and cucumber sticks. Hummus, made from chickpeas, offers fiber and protein, while the crunchy vegetables provide hydration and additional fiber.

Another super easy recipe is chia seed pudding with coconut milk, a tasty treat that requires minimal effort. Chia seeds are packed with fiber and omega-3 fatty acids, which can help reduce inflammation and support gut health. Simply mix chia seeds with coconut milk and let them soak overnight. By morning, you'll have a pudding-like consistency that can be flavored with a hint of vanilla or topped with your favorite berries. Another homemade option is roasted chickpeas with cumin and paprika. These little morsels are packed with fiber and protein, offering a satisfying crunch that mimics the texture of less healthy snacks like chips. Roasting chickpeas with spices makes them more delicious and adds anti-inflammatory benefits, making them a perfect savory snack.

When you're out and about, choosing gut-friendly snacks can be at times more challenging, but not impossible. Start by reading labels carefully, checking the fiber content. Fiber is your friend when it comes to staying full and keeping your digestive system happy. Aim for snacks with whole food ingredients, avoiding those with artificial additives or excessive sugars. Choose snacks that are minimally processed and have natural ingredients. Nuts and seeds, for example, are excellent on-the-go options. They're not only portable but also rich in healthy fats and fiber, making them ideal for supporting gut health even when you're miles from your kitchen.

Snacking is often considered a guilty pleasure, but it doesn't have to be. By making mindful choices, you can turn each snack into an opportunity to nourish your body and support your gut health.

REFRESHING BEVERAGES FOR GUT BALANCE

While food often takes center stage in discussions about digestion, the drinks you choose can also have a huge impact on maintaining hydration and digestive balance. Hydration is key for digestion; it helps break down food, allowing nutrients to be absorbed more efficiently. When you're well-hydrated, your gut can function more smoothly, reducing the risk of constipation and other digestive discomforts.

Certain ingredients in beverages can also boost their gut-friendly qualities. Herbal teas like peppermint and chamomile are excellent choices. Peppermint tea is known for its soothing effects on the digestive tract, helping to relieve bloating and gas. Chamomile, on the other hand, is a gentle relaxant that can calm the digestive system and reduce inflammation. Both offer more than just hydration; they provide therapeutic benefits that support overall gut health. Lemon water with a dash of apple cider vinegar is another simple yet powerful drink. Lemon adds vitamin C and a refreshing zing, while apple cider vinegar is thought to help with digestion by promoting the production of stomach acid. These ingredients work in harmony, offering a refreshing way to support your digestive system.

Consider starting your day with a glass of lemon water. It's a simple ritual that can kickstart digestion and hydrate your body after a night's rest.

Why not try a steaming cup of ginger and turmeric tea? This beverage harnesses the anti-inflammatory properties of both ingredients, helping to soothe the digestive tract and reduce discomfort. To make it, simply boil slices of fresh ginger and a teaspoon of turmeric in water, allowing the flavors to meld before straining into a cup. So easy!

For something colder, try a kefir smoothie with mixed berries. Kefir is a fermented drink rich in probiotics, which aid in maintaining a healthy gut flora. Blending it with berries adds antioxidants and fiber.

Adding these easy, healthy drinks into your daily routine can become a nourishing habit.

PREPARING MEALS FOR GUT HEALTH ON-THE-GO

I know that trying to look after your gut and general health with a busy lifestyle or while traveling often poses unique challenges. It's not easy! When facing unhealthy choices at every turn and limited access to nutritious meal options (or overpriced healthy options), it's tempting to grab whatever's convenient, even if it doesn't serve your gut well. Fast food joints and processed snacks are everywhere, but they rarely offer the fiber and nutrients your gut craves. Not only that, you can feel sluggish on a trip when you need energy more than ever. It might feel like an uphill battle, but with a little planning, you can arm yourself with gut-friendly meals that don't compromise on convenience or taste.

Packing portable snacks is your first line of defense. Nuts and seeds are excellent choices, packed with fiber and healthy fats that keep you satisfied and your digestion in check. They're easy to stash in your bag, requiring no refrigeration or special prep. For something heartier, prepare meals at home using insulated containers. These handy tools keep your food fresh and ready to eat when you need a nourishing break. They're truly your secret weapon against the lure of fast food, allowing you to enjoy a homemade meal no matter where you are.

You could try making a quinoa salad with chickpeas and cherry tomatoes before your next trip or a busy day. Quinoa is a complete protein, and chickpeas provide additional fiber and protein. The cherry tomatoes add a burst of color and flavor, making this salad both visually appealing and delicious. It's a simple dish that holds up well in transit, ensuring you have a satisfying, gut-friendly option ready whenever hunger strikes. For a more substantial meal, try whole grain wraps with turkey and avocado. The whole grains provide the necessary fiber, the turkey offers lean protein, and the avocado brings in healthy fats, creating a balanced meal that supports your digestive health.

Dining out while trying to maintain gut health can also be tricky, but not impossible. One effective strategy is to opt for dishes that feature whole grains and plenty of vegetables. These ingredients are more likely to support your digestion and overall health and keep your energy levels up when you're on the go. When scanning the menu, don't hesitate to ask for dressings and sauces on the side. This simple request allows you to control the amount you consume, reducing unnecessary fats and sugars that might otherwise sneak into your meal. It's a small adjustment that can make a big difference in how your gut feels afterward.

As we move forward, we will look at how you can continue to nurture your gut through mindful lifestyle choices and habits.

CONCLUSION

As we come to the end of this book, I want to take a moment to contemplate together the fabulous path we've walked. We've studied the fascinating world of gut health, identifying the intricate connections between our digestive system and overall well-being. We've learned that by taking care of our gut and giving it our time and attention, we can unleash a vibrant, energized version of ourselves, ready to take on the world!

Let's recap the key insights we've discovered. We now understand that the gut is a digestive organ but also a complex ecosystem that influences every aspect of our health. By working on creating a diverse, balanced microbiome through nourishing foods and mindful lifestyle choices, we can do so much to support our gut's natural ability to thrive! We've seen how simple practices like adding prebiotics and probiotics, prioritizing fiber-rich meals, and managing stress can have an amazing immediate and long-term impact on our digestive harmony.

But knowledge alone isn't enough; it's time to put these insights into action! Start small, perhaps by adding a probiotic-rich food to your daily routine or taking a few minutes to practice deep breathing exercises. Remember, every choice you make, no matter how small, is a step towards a healthier, happier gut. As you continue to implement these changes, you'll begin to feel the transformative effects ripple through your body and mind, and I'm sure you'll be keen to add more and more healthy changes.

This is just the beginning. Enjoy the ongoing process of learning, experimenting, and adapting. Stay curious about the latest research and innovations in gut health, and don't be afraid to try new things and ask for help when unsure or in need of a professional, guiding hand. Your body is unique, and what works for someone else might not work for you. Trust your instincts, listen to your gut (literally!), and keep refining your approach.

And remember, you're not alone! You're part of a growing community of individuals who are prioritizing their gut health and, in turn, transforming their lives. Lean on this community for support, inspiration, and encouragement. Share your experiences, celebrate your successes, and learn from others who are on a similar path.

I want to express my heartfelt gratitude for your commitment to this process. By picking up this book and dedicating yourself to understanding your gut, you've taken a massive step towards reclaiming your health. Your determination and openness to change are genuinely inspiring, and I have no doubt that you'll continue to make incredible strides in your wellness journey.

Your gut health is a lifelong journey, and I'm honored to have been a part of it! Now, go forth with confidence, knowing that every step you take is leading you toward a brighter, healthier future. Your best self is waiting; let's go meet them!

SELF HEALTH GUT GUIDE BONUS QUESTIONS

Congratulations on reaching this pivotal point in your gut health journey! By throwing yourself into the pages of this book, you've already begun a transformative path toward understanding the unique language of your body. This is no small feat, and you should really celebrate the progress you've made.

I created this section because I understand that everyone connects and reflects in their own unique way. Sometimes, a single question might not resonate, and that's perfectly okay. Sometimes, it takes asking a different question or exploring an idea from another angle to truly spark clarity. That's why I've crafted this space for additional exploration, designed to enrich your experience even further. If you're feeling curious and eager to dive a little deeper, this toolkit of thoughtful prompts is here for you whenever you're ready. These questions are broken up by chapters and are meant to gently encourage you to pause, reflect, and peel back more layers of understanding—all at your own comfortable pace.

So, allow yourself the freedom to examine different angles and connect more deeply with your well-being. You have the knowledge, and now it's time to trust your intuition to lead the way.

Introduction

Self-Reflection on Symptoms

- What are some symptoms or discomforts you've been experiencing that might signal an imbalance in your gut health?
- How long have you been noticing these symptoms?

Emotional Connection

- How do you feel emotionally when you experience these symptoms?
- Do any emotions or feelings typically accompany your physical symptoms?

Envisioning the Future

- Imagine a future where your gut health is balanced and thriving.
- How do you envision your life and daily experiences changing as a result?

Personalized Approach

- Recognizing that a one-size-fits-all approach doesn't work, how comfortable are you with experimenting and making adjustments to your routine to discover what truly benefits you?

Chapter 1

Your Gut Ecosystem: Balance and Diversity

- How comfortable are you with trying new foods that could enhance your gut health, such as fermented foods or a broader range of fiber-rich options?

The Microbiome Revolution

- What aspects of your current lifestyle might be impacting your gut microbiome positively or negatively?
- Consider a time when you noticed a change in your health or mood that may have been related to your diet. What different choices might have changed that outcome?
- How do you balance the need for occasional medication, such as antibiotics, with the goal of maintaining a healthy microbiome?

Gut-Brain Axis: The Fascinating Mind-Gut Connection

- Reflect on a situation where you felt a 'gut feeling' about something. How did you react, and what was the outcome?
- How might understanding the gut-brain connection change your perspective towards addressing mental health issues?
- What steps can you take to nurture both your mind and gut through diet and lifestyle?

Gut Health: Your Immune System's Secret Weapon

- Consider your current habits. How do they potentially support or suppress your immune system?
- What is one new habit you're willing to try out, such as consuming more probiotics, to boost your immune health?
- How aware are you of the role your gut health plays in your body's response to vaccines and infections?

Red Flags: Signs of Gut Imbalance

- What subtle signals has your body been sending you about your gut health that you might have overlooked?
- Have you ever tried tracking your food intake and symptoms? If not, what's preventing you from starting a journal now?
- If you experience unexplained symptoms, what practical steps can you take to seek advice and support for addressing potential gut health issues?

The Science of Gut Health: Foundations and Facts

- Given what you've learned, does any gut health myth you previously believed about gut health surprise you now?
- How might the future possibilities of personalized nutrition excite or worry you?

Chapter 2

Fueling Your Gut with Probiotics and Prebiotics

- Consider a day without access to specific foods. What are some alternative sources of probiotics or prebiotics that you can include in your daily diet to ensure continuous gut support?

Plant-Based Power: Fiber for a Healthy Gut

- What current role does fiber play in your diet? How might you creatively incorporate more fiber without completely altering your favorite dishes?
- Do you currently experience any digestive discomfort? How might increasing fiber in your diet impact these feelings, and what steps will you take to ensure a gentle transition?
- How can you make meal planning an engaging and fun process to experiment with new fiber-rich recipes?

Anti-Inflammatory Foods

- Take stock of the inflammatory foods you commonly consume. What are some practical steps you can take to gradually replace these with anti-inflammatory alternatives?
- Reflect on how your body feels after consuming certain anti-inflammatory foods like turmeric or omega-3-rich fish. What differences do you notice in your gut health and overall vitality?
- What new anti-inflammatory food will you try this week, and how will you incorporate it into your meals?

Fabulous Fermented Foods: Natural (and Delicious!) Probiotic Sources

- If you're new to fermented foods, which one are you most excited to try and why? How do you plan to incorporate it into your diet?
- When exploring new fermented foods, consider any hesitations or concerns you might have. How can you ease into trying and enjoying these novel flavors and textures?

Creating a Gut-Friendly Meal Plan

- How can you balance meal prep with a busy schedule to ensure that maintaining a gut-friendly diet remains a priority?
- Reflect on the variety of foods you consume. Are there any food groups you're neglecting? How can you bring more diversity into your diet?
- How does meal planning assist you in making better dietary decisions, and what new strategies will you adopt to enhance this process?

Eating Your Way: Dietary Needs & Preferences

- Consider your current dietary restrictions. How have you adapted to ensure you still consume a nutritious, balanced diet that supports your gut health?
- How do you view eating out with dietary restrictions? What strategies will you use to feel confident and informed when dining at restaurants or social gatherings?

- Reflect on how your perspective towards dietary restrictions has evolved. In what ways have you embraced a mindset that focuses on possibilities and new experiences?

Chapter 3

Stress and Gut Health

- Consider the stress management techniques you currently use. Which new practices will you try to alleviate stress and its impact on your gut?
- Reflect on a recent stressful situation. How did it affect your body, and what could you have done to mitigate its impact?

Sleep and Digestion: The Secret to a Restored Body

- Analyze your current sleep routine. How might disruptions in sleep be affecting your digestion and overall gut health?
- Reflect on the changes you could implement to improve your sleep hygiene. What has prevented you from establishing these habits in the past?

Movement and Microbiota: Get Moving for Your Gut

- How does your current exercise routine support or hinder your gut health?
- What types of physical activities appeal to you most, and how can you incorporate them into your routine to benefit your gut?

- Reflect on how you can introduce more movement into your daily life, even in small, manageable ways.

Mindful Eating: How Awareness Nourishes Your Gut

- How often do you practice mindful eating? What barriers prevent you from being fully present during meals?
- Reflect on a recent meal. How did practicing mindfulness affect your eating experience and digestive wellness?
- What steps can you take to make mindful eating a consistent part of your routine?

Building a Happy Gut: Look Around You

- Examine your living environment. What changes can you make to reduce exposure to toxins and create a more gut-friendly space?
- Reflect on the household products you currently use. How can switching to natural alternatives benefit your health?

Stronger Together: How Community Boosts Your Health

- How strong are your social connections, and how might they impact your gut health?
- Are there any relationships or friendships that may not be good for you? For example, could you be in a toxic friendship/relationship? If so, it may be significantly affecting your physical and mental health. Consider if they are supporting you or draining you. Nudging you forward, or holding you back.

- Reflect on the balance between social interaction and solitude in your life. How can you build a healthier balance to benefit your mind and gut?

Chapter 4
Bloating and Gas: Tackling Common Digestive Discomforts

- Reflect on recent instances when you've experienced bloating or gas. What might have triggered these symptoms, and how did they affect your daily activities?
- What role do you think your gut microbiome plays in these digestive issues, and what steps can you take to support a healthier balance?

Leaky Gut: Understanding and Healing

- Based on what you've learned, what lifestyle factors might contribute to increased gut permeability in your case?
- What dietary changes can you implement to support gut lining repair and reduce inflammation?
- How might stress management play a role in healing a leaky gut, and what specific techniques will you integrate into your routine?

Food Sensitivities and Allergies: Discovering What Works for You

- Have you suspected any food sensitivities or allergies? What steps will you take to identify and manage them effectively?

- How has food affected you physically and emotionally, and how can keeping a food journal aid in detecting sensitivities?
- What plan will you establish to ensure you receive adequate nutrition while avoiding triggers due to food sensitivities or allergies?

The Role of Antibiotics and Gut Recovery

- Have you recently used antibiotics? How can you facilitate your gut's recovery post-treatment?
- What strategies can you adopt to limit your antibiotic use, ensuring it's only employed when necessary?
- How can maintaining a balanced gut microbiome aid in reducing the need for antibiotics over time?

Gut Health in the Modern World: Balancing Wellness with Life's Demands

- How does your current lifestyle, including work, stress level, and screen time, impact your gut health?
- What small changes can you make to your daily routine to better support your gut amidst your busy schedule?
- Can you identify ways to disconnect from technology to better align yourself with your body's natural rhythms?

Trusting the Process: Overcoming Doubts on Your Gut Health Journey

- What gut health practices currently resonate with you, and how will you ensure they're rooted in evidence-based information?

- How can you personalize your approach to gut health, aligning dietary and lifestyle choices with your unique needs?

Chapter 5

Personal Triggers and Reactions

- What foods have you discovered trigger reactions in your body?
- How have you confirmed these triggers through journaling or self-assessment tools?

Goal Setting and Tracking Progress

- What are one short-term and one long-term goal you can set for improving your gut health? How can you make these goals SMART (Specific, Measurable, Achievable, Relevant, Time-bound)?
- Reflect on a previous goal you set and achieved. What was key to your success, and how can you apply those lessons to your gut health journey?

Integrative Wellness Approach

- How do your current fitness and wellness routines support your gut health? What additional practices could enhance this partnership?
- How can you incorporate mindfulness or community activities into your routine to support both mental health and gut wellness?

Chapter 6

Cultural Practices and Personal Exploration

- What cultural food traditions resonate most with you? How might they inspire changes in your dietary habits to promote better gut health?

Innovations and Future Insights

- Which recent advancements in gut health research intrigue you the most? How can you apply this knowledge to your current approach to health?
- Consider the potential benefits and challenges of personalized nutrition. How open are you to trying new technologies or dietary strategies that promise customized health solutions?

Challenging Myths

- Have you subscribed to any gut health myths or misconceptions in the past? What experiences or new information have led you to question or reject these?
- How do you evaluate health information? What criteria do you use to determine if a source is credible?

Genetic Influences

- How might your family history influence your approach to gut health? Consider any digestive issues or conditions that are common in your family.
- What steps can you take to learn more about how your

genetic makeup might affect your digestion and overall health?

Chapter 7

Breakfast Transformations

- Reflect on your current breakfast habits. How can you incorporate more fiber and probiotics to boost your morning routine?

Balanced Lunches

- Analyze your typical lunch. Is it balanced with fiber, protein, and healthy fats?
- What simple changes can you make to improve its gut health value? Are there new foods you'd be willing to try?

Dinner Decisions

- What are your dinner staples, and how do they support or hinder your gut health? Are there particular legumes or grains you'd like to experiment with?
- How do your evening meal choices impact your sleep quality and late-night cravings?

Smart Snacking

- Reflect on your snacking habits. Do they contribute positively to your gut health? What swaps can you make for more nourishing snacks?
- How do you plan your snacks when you're out or traveling? What strategies could make this easier?

Mindful Beverages

- Consider your current beverage choices. Which drinks could you add to your routine to enhance hydration and support digestion?
- Reflect on how herbal teas and probiotic-rich drinks make you feel compared to sugary or caffeinated alternatives.

On-the-Go Preparedness

- What challenges do you face when trying to eat healthily on the go? How can you prepare to overcome these obstacles?
- Reflect on the last time you traveled. What worked well for maintaining gut health, and where could you improve?

Self Health Gut Guide RESOURCE GUIDE

I'm excited to share with you a handpicked collection of resources that have been valuable on my own self health and gut health journey. In this section, I'll share with you a wealth of knowledge from diverse sources, including insightful websites and knowledgeable providers who offer a deeper understanding of gut health. I've also included talented recipe developers who create delicious and gut-friendly meals to further inspire your kitchen adventures. You'll find handy apps for tracking your progress and some interesting podcasts that provide thought-provoking discussions. These resources have supported and guided me along the way, and I hope they offer you the same encouragement and enlightenment as you continue your personal path to vibrant health. Remember, the journey is all about listening to your body and finding what resonates with you. Enjoy checking out these wonderful tools!

1. Websites and Online Communities: Stay updated on the latest gut health information from reputable sources.

General Health Websites with Comprehensive Gut Health Information:

- **Mayo Clinic:** A leading source for general health information, including a dedicated section on digestive health and conditions like IBS.
- **WebMD:** Offers a wide range of health topics, with detailed information on gut health, symptoms, causes, and treatment options.
- **National Institutes of Health (NIH) MedlinePlus:** Provides reliable, consumer-friendly information on various health topics, including gut health, based on peer-reviewed research.

Specialized Gut Health Websites and Forums:

- **The Gut Health Clinic:** Run by a team of digestive health specialists, offering articles, blog posts, and educational videos on various aspects of gut health.
- **Gut Health Support Group:** An online forum where individuals with gut health issues can connect, share experiences, and offer support to one another.
- **Crohn's & Colitis Foundation:** A leading organization dedicated to Crohn's disease and ulcerative colitis, providing information, resources, and support for patients.

Important Considerations When Evaluating Online Sources:

- **Credibility:** Check for credentials and affiliations of the website authors. Look for sources backed by scientific research institutions, registered healthcare professionals, or established organizations.
- **Accuracy:** Verify information against reputable sources like those listed above. Be wary of sensationalized claims or unsubstantiated advice.
- **Community Guidelines:** When participating in online forums, be mindful of respectful communication and avoid sharing personal medical advice without consulting a healthcare professional.

Tip: When seeking information online, discuss it with your healthcare provider to ensure it aligns with your individual needs and health conditions.

2. Podcasts and Videos: Recommended podcasts or YouTube channels that frequently feature experts discussing gut health topics.

- **"The Gut Health Gurus Podcast"** delivers easy-to-digest tips and expert advice on boosting your gut health naturally.
- **"The Doctor's Farmacy"** hosted by Dr. Mark Hyman, explores holistic health, including gut health.
- YouTube channel **NutritionFacts.org** by Dr. Michael Greger for science-based nutrition facts.
- **"Gut Health Reset with Dr. Ann-Marie Barter"** discusses issues that start in the gut and offers insights and strategies to improve digestive health and overall well-being.

- **"The Wellness Mama Podcast"** which covers a variety of health topics, including gut health.
- **TED Talks** on gut health and the microbiome, such as those by Rob Knight.

3. Professionals and Experts: List of nutritionists, dietitians, and holistic health practitioners who specialize in gut health or have resourceful websites to gain more knowledge from.

- **The Institute for Functional Medicine's** practitioner directory to find experts who specialize in gut health.
- Websites like **Zocdoc** or **Healthgrades** often feature profiles of nutritionists and dietitians offering telehealth services.
- **The British Dietetic Association's** directory for registered dietitians.
- Listings on **Telehealth.org** to find specialists offering remote consultations.
- **Dr. Deanna Minich** focuses on color and diverse foods to empower individuals to achieve vibrant health. Offers many free downloads, such as a food/mood weekly tracker.
- **The Gut Health Doctor** whose expert guidance and practical tips on improving gut health through science-backed nutrition and lifestyle strategies.

4. Recipes and Meal Plans: Suggestions for finding gut-friendly recipes and meal plans.

- **Minimalist Baker** has easy-to-follow recipes that typically require ten ingredients or less, one bowl, or

thirty minutes or less to prepare, focusing on simplicity and flavor for everyday cooking
- Utilize the website **EatRight.org** for nutritionally sound meal planning.
- **"Deliciously Ella's Plant-Based Cookbook"** by Ella Woodward, which includes gut-friendly recipes and the **Deliciously Ella app** for recipes, shopping lists, and balanced meal plans that help you get diversity in your diet.
- **Eating Well** features recipes that are often created or reviewed by registered dietitians or nutrition experts, including gut health diet.
- Websites like **SIBOinfo.com** provide meal plans specifically for small intestinal bacterial overgrowth.
- **BBC Good Food** provides recipes tagged for gut health.

Here are some of my favorite sites for discovering healthy, veggie-loaded recipes that boost your food diversity and fiber intake with meals rich in plant-based ingredients. Browsing these sites can inspire some new and delicious ways to incorporate more plants into your meals, whether you're fully committed to a plant-based diet or looking to complement your meals that include meat.

- **The Natural Nurturer**
- **Minimalist Baker**
- **Dishing Up the Dirt**
- **Oh She Glows**
- **Dishing Out the Health**

5. Supplements and Products: How to choose quality options with so many supplements to choose from these days.

Important Note: *I always recommend consulting with a healthcare provider before starting any supplement regimen*

Exploring the Supplement Aisle

Selecting a high-quality supplement can be tricky. Educating yourself as a consumer and understanding how to recognize premium supplements is advantageous for both coaches and their clients. The FDA has established a few guidelines that manufacturers should adhere to, including ensuring the safety of their products, making truthful claims, and following the Federal Food, Drug, and Cosmetic Act along with FDA regulations. Additionally, all supplements should be produced in facilities that observe good manufacturing practices (GMP certification).

Nevertheless, it's ultimately the manufacturers' responsibility to follow these guidelines. In the U.S., the FDA neither tests nor approves dietary supplements. As such, consider the following when evaluating supplements:

- **Sourcing**: Opt for brands that are transparent about their ingredient list and their origins.
- **Additives and Fillers**: Steer clear of excessive ingredients that could introduce toxins or trigger adverse reactions.
- **Testing**: Some products are tested by third-party organizations like USP Verified or NSF International. Look for these certifications.
- **Effectiveness**: Supplements should be efficient and easily absorbed. Confirm if any vitamins need to be paired with other nutrients to work effectively and ensure the supplement hasn't expired.
- **Research**: Investigate whether companies offer clinical studies or general research, and check if they collaborate with scientific or medical experts.

6. Apps for Tracking and Management: Apps that can help track gut health, diet, and lifestyle changes.

- The **Deliciously Ella** app has wellness tracking, including sleep, movement, mindfulness, food diversity, and hydration.
- **Cara Care** and **MySymptoms** are apps designed to track symptoms, diet, and gut health-related moods.
- **Yazio** for comprehensive diet tracking with a focus on gut-friendly foods.
- **Ate Visual Food Journal and Diary** for mindful and intuitive eating journaling.

7. Mindfulness, Movement, and Stress-Reduction Resources: Since stress can impact gut health, here are some resources for yoga, meditation, or other stress-reduction techniques.

- **Headspace** and **Calm** apps for guided meditation.
- YouTube has excellent yoga resources, like **Yoga with Adriene**.
- Articles on mindfulness practices from **Mindful.org**.
- **Insight Timer** app for meditation.
- **10% Happier** for practical mindfulness strategies.
- **Deliciously Ella** app for wellness classes - barre, yoga, cardio, and Pilates.
- The **Nike Training** app has many workout and mindset options, such as breathing exercises.
- **Jillian Michaels** app provides a selection of movement and mindfulness choices, plus more, such as a community and support.

REFERENCES

The role of gut microbiota in immune homeostasis and ... (n.d.). PubMed Central. https://pmc.ncbi.nlm.nih.gov/articles/PMC3337124/

Role of diet and its effects on the gut microbiome ... (2022). Nature. https://www.nature.com/articles/s41398-022-01922-0

The gut-brain axis: interactions between enteric microbiota, ... (n.d.). PubMed Central. https://pmc.ncbi.nlm.nih.gov/articles/PMC4367209/

Gut Microbiota and Immune System Interactions. (n.d.). PubMed Central. https://pmc.ncbi.nlm.nih.gov/articles/PMC7602490/

Probiotics and prebiotics: What you should know. (n.d.). Mayo Clinic. https://www.mayoclinic.org/healthy-lifestyle/nutrition-and-healthy-eating/expert-answers/probiotics/faq-20058065#:~:text=Probiotics%20are%20foods%20or%20supplements,as%20food%20for%20human%20microflora.

22 High-Fiber Foods You Should Eat. (n.d.). Healthline. https://www.healthline.com/nutrition/22-high-fiber-foods

Anti-Inflammatory Eating for Gut Health: Connecting Diet ... (n.d.). Rupa Health. https://www.rupahealth.com/post/anti-inflammatory-eating-for-gut-health-connecting-diet-and-digestion

Fermented-food diet increases microbiome diversity ... (2021). Stanford Medicine News. https://med.stanford.edu/news/all-news/2021/07/fermented-food-diet-increases-microbiome-diversity-lowers-inflammation.html

How Cortisol Affects Gut Health & The Microbiome. (n.d.). The Beauty Chef. https://thebeautychef.com/blogs/articles/how-cortisol-affects-gut-health-and-the-microbiome?srsltid=AfmBOorn-Lb03OMDtsqKgdjxk6QV1CuYkH2qJGf98kWV3EXI1V-PT2gb

The gut microbiota, HPA axis, and brain in adolescent-onset ... (n.d.). ScienceDirect. https://www.sciencedirect.com/science/article/pii/S2666354622001314#:~:text=HPA%2Daxis%20activation%20by%20stress,2018%3B%20Galley%20et%20al.%2C

Exercise Modifies the Gut Microbiota with Positive ... (n.d.). PubMed Central. https://pmc.ncbi.nlm.nih.gov/articles/PMC5357536/

Mindful Eating. (n.d.). Harvard Health Publications. https://www.health.harvard.edu/staying-healthy/mindful-eating

FODMAP Diet 101: A Detailed Beginner's Guide. (n.d.). Healthline. https://www.healthline.com/nutrition/fodmaps-101

Leaky Gut Syndrome: Myths and Management. (n.d.). PubMed Central. https://pmc.ncbi.nlm.nih.gov/articles/PMC11345991/

Food Allergy vs. Intolerance: What's the Difference? (n.d.). Cleveland Clinic Health Essentials. https://health.clevelandclinic.org/allergy-or-intolerance-how-to-tell-the-difference

Recovery of gut microbiota of healthy adults following ... (2018). Nature. https://www.nature.com/articles/s41564-018-0257-9

What to know about microbiome testing. (n.d.). Medical News Today. https://www.medicalnewstoday.com/articles/microbiome-testing

Be SMART about setting health-related goals | Diet and Nutrition. (n.d.). UT Southwestern Medical Center. https://utswmed.org/medblog/smart-goals-health-wellness/

Best Gut Health Apps of 2020. (n.d.). Healthline. https://www.healthline.com/health/digestive-health/top-iphone-android-apps-gut-health

Systematic analysis of gut microbiota in pregnant women ... (2020). Nature. https://www.nature.com/articles/s41522-020-00142-y

Diet and the Human Gut Microbiome. (n.d.). PubMed Central. https://pmc.ncbi.nlm.nih.gov/articles/PMC7117800/

Gut microbiome in 2023: current and emerging research ... (n.d.). Gut Microbiota for Health. https://www.gutmicrobiotaforhealth.com/gut-microbiome-in-2023-current-and-emerging-research-trends/

10 Gut Myths, Corrected. (2025, January 22). The New York Times. https://www.nytimes.com/2025/01/22/well/gut-health-myths.html

Human Genetics Shape the Gut Microbiome. (n.d.). Cell. https://www.cell.com/fulltext/S0092-8674(14)01241-0

The #1 Breakfast for Gut Health, Recommended by ... (n.d.). EatingWell. https://www.eatingwell.com/article/8062398/best-breakfast-for-gut-health/

Dietary fiber: Essential for a healthy diet. (n.d.). Mayo Clinic. https://www.mayoclinic.org/healthy-lifestyle/nutrition-and-healthy-eating/in-depth/fiber/art-20043983

25 Gut-Healthy Lunches That Are High in Protein. (n.d.). EatingWell. https://www.eatingwell.com/gut-healthy-high-protein-lunch-recipes-8636200

Anti-inflammatory diet meal plan: 26 healthful recipes. (n.d.). Medical News Today. https://www.medicalnewstoday.com/articles/322897

Designing Interactive Experiences For Gut Health ... (n.d.). ResearchGate. https://www.researchgate.net/publication/370173307_Designing_Interactive_Experiences_For_Gut_Health_Engagement_and_Reflection

How to boost your wellbeing – the benefits of a growth mindset. (n.d.). ThinkWell Psychology. https://www.thinkwellpsychology.com.au/news/how-to-boost-your-wellbeing-the-benefits-of-a-growth-mindset

6 Inspirational Medical Stories of Patient Perseverance and ... (n.d.). Johnson &

Johnson. https://www.jnj.com/personal-stories/6-inspirational-medical-stories-of-patient-perseverance-and-resilience

OpenAI. (2023). ChatGPT [Large language model]. Retrieved from https://chat.openai.com/

New computational tool accurately assesses health ... (2020, September 3). News-Medical. https://www.news-medical.net/news/20240903/New-computational-tool-accurately-assesses-health-through-gut-microbiome-analysis.aspx

Printed in Dunstable, United Kingdom